教育部生物医学工程类专业教学指导委员会"十三五"规划教材

生物医学工程专业英语

刘　蓉　齐莉萍　编著

U0294100

电子工业出版社
Publishing House of Electronics Industry
北京 · BEIJING

内 容 简 介

全书共有 12 个单元（unit），每个单元均包含 text、listening、writing、speaking 四个部分。内容涵盖生物医学工程、基因和生物信息学、解剖学和生理学、生物材料、组织工程、生物力学、康复工程、生物医学传感器、生物信号处理、生物医学仪器、医学影像、道德与伦理等。内容选材新、知识面广、难度适中，并配有听力音频文件。

本书可供普通高等学校生物医学工程专业的本科生及研究生作为专业英语教材，也可作为相关工程技术人员学习专业英语的参考用书。

图书在版编目（CIP）数据

生物医学工程专业英语 / 刘蓉，齐莉萍编著. —北京：电子工业出版社，2020.5（2025.3 重印）
ISBN 978-7-121-37053-3

Ⅰ. ①生… Ⅱ. ①刘… ②齐… Ⅲ. ①生物工程－医学工程－英语－高等学校－教材 Ⅳ. ①R318

中国版本图书馆 CIP 数据核字（2019）第 140117 号

责任编辑：张小乐 特约编辑：邢彤彤
印　　刷：北京虎彩文化传播有限公司
装　　订：北京虎彩文化传播有限公司
出版发行：电子工业出版社
　　　　　北京市海淀区万寿路 173 信箱　　邮编：100036
开　　本：787×1 092　1/16　印张：9.25　字数：308 千字
版　　次：2020 年 5 月第 1 版
印　　次：2025 年 3 月第 9 次印刷
定　　价：32.00 元

教育部生物医学工程类专业教学指导委员会
"十三五"规划教材编审委员会

总　序

　　生物医学工程（Biomedical Engineering，BME）是运用工程学的原理和方法解决生物医学问题，提高人类健康水平的综合性学科。它在生物学与医学领域融合数学、物理、化学、信息和计算机科学，运用工程学的原理与方法获取和产生新知识，创造新方法，从分子、细胞、组织、器官、生命系统各层面丰富生命科学的知识宝库，推动生命科学的研究进程，促进生命科学和医疗卫生事业的发展，实现提高人类健康水平的伟大使命。

　　现代生物医学工程以 1952 年美国无线电工程学会（Institute of Radio Engineers，IRE）成立的医学电子学专业组（Professional Group on Medical Electronics，PGME）为标志，经过近 70 年的发展已成为一个学科涵盖面最广的专业。**多学科融合是生物医学工程类专业的特质**，其包含的主要领域有：生物医学电子学，生物医学光子学，生物医学仪器，医学成像，医学材料，生物生物力学，生物医学信息学，仿生学，细胞、组织和基因工程，临床工程，矫形工程，康复工程，神经工程，系统生理学，生物医学纳米技术，医学监督和管理，医学培训和教育等。

　　"十三五"期间，国家发布了"健康中国 2030"规划纲要，提出"要将人民健康放在优先发展的战略地位"。与此相关的生物医学工程在国家发展和经济建设中具有重要的战略地位，是医疗健康事业发展的重要基础和推动引擎。生物医学工程所涉及的医学仪器、医学材料等是世界上发展最迅速的支柱性产业，已成为国家科技水平和核心竞争力的重要标志，是国家经济建设中优先发展的重要领域。

　　生物医学工程事业发展需要大量专业人才。我国的生物医学工程高等教育始于 20 世纪 70 年代中后期，经过 40 多年的发展，全国设置 BME 专业的高校已达 180 余所。为了适应科技和教育发展的需要，教育部高等学校生物医学工程类专业教学指导委员会（下简称"教指委"）与电子工业出版社经过深入调研，精心设计，成立了生物医学工程类专业"十三五"规划教材编审委员会，启动了规划教材建设项目。项目汇集了一批兼具丰富教学和科研经验的专家学者，经广泛研讨，编著了符合《生物医学工程类专业教学质量国家标准》的数十部教材，涵盖医学信号与图像、医学电子、医学仪器、生物医学传感与检测、医学统计与临床实验、生物医学工程伦理等重要课程和领域。规划教材充分体现生物医学工程类专业多学科融合的特质，深浅适度，阐明原理并列举典型应用实例。规划教材还特别设立了"康复科学与技术"系列，以满足康复工程专业人才培养的迫切要求，助力我国康复事业的发展。

　　教指委和规划教材编审委员会感谢各位专家给予的支持和帮助！感谢所有参与编著的学者！希望这套教材能让学生热爱生物医学工程，并扎根于此。

　　恳切希望读者能对这套教材的不足之处提出宝贵意见和建议，以便再版时更正。

生物医学工程学类专业教指委
"十三五"规划教材编审委员会
2020 年 3 月

前　言

编者在大连理工大学生物医学工程学院教授"科技英语"课程期间，通过与学生进行课堂互动提问，以及交流学习英语的心得与经验，发现学生用英语进行交流有很好的基础，并对能够用英语自如地交流抱有很高的期望。尝试在教学环节中增加英语的应用技巧训练后，发现学生能够更迅速地掌握英语表达的要领，并有条不紊地演练、准备，在实践中表现得更为自信。

基于在教学实践中积累的一些思考、尝试和体会，我们编写了本书，力求帮助学生从听、说、读、写四个方面着手对英语应用能力的培养。目前大多数关于科技英语的教材依然以科技文献的阅读理解为主，让学生常常误认为科技英语是以知识为导向的课程。然而，随着国际科技文化交流日益频繁，本科生、研究生参与科研、撰写科研论文以及参加国际会议的机会不断增加，需要将更有针对性的英语应用能力和技巧加以补充。本书的编写，以科技英语的应用实践为目的，让学生能够均衡地提高听、说、读、写方面的能力，并着重演练英文科技论文写作、国际会议口头报告的能力。

全书共有 12 个单元（unit），每个单元均包含 text、listening、writing、speaking 四部分。每个单元的阅读材料对应生物医学工程领域的一个分支，学生可以将其与专业课所学知识相结合，作为有益的扩展和补充。在阅读部分还提供了专业词汇与翻译的资料库，以帮助学生增强对相关知识的理解，进而有效地应用到阅读与翻译中。听力训练的内容取材于维基百科和 *Nature*、*Science*、*Cell* 等知名期刊，与阅读材料相互呼应、相辅相成。听力录音由加拿大语言学博士 Artur Bohnet 录制。听力材料可作为反复跟读和复述的范本。写作部分梳理总结了英语科技论文的写作规范、技能和实例，将完整的科技论文拆分开进行细致的讲解，并附有写作模板与练习。口语部分主要针对国际性学术会议报告所需的综合能力，包括会议报告PPT 的组织架构、各部分的主要内容及各个部分之间的衔接与过渡，鼓励学生创新性地表达专业思想。此外，书中还整理了会议报告常用句型和演讲技巧。

在教学实践中的探索与尝试，令我们受益匪浅。通过课堂上与学生进行英语交流，不断深化对科技英语教学与实践的认识，梳理自身的知识体系，继而完善教学内容。深知英语应用能力的提高绝非短短的课程能够实现的，希望学生以此教材中所列的内容为基础，在应用英语的过程中，不断实践、不断完善、主动学习、终身学习。

由于时间和编者水平有限，书中错漏与不足之处在所难免，敬请读者批评指正。

编　者
2019 年 7 月于大连

目　　录

Unit 1　Biomedical Engineering

1.1　Text: Biomedical Engineering

Many of the problems the health professionals confronting today are of extreme importance to the engineer because they involve the fundamental aspects of device and systems analysis, design, and practical application—all of which lie at the heart of processes that are fundamental to engineering practice.[1] These medically relevant design problems can range from very complex large-scale constructs, such as the design and implementation of automated clinical laboratories, multiphasic screening facilities (i.e. centers that permit many tests to be conducted), and hospital information systems, to the creation of relatively small and simple devices, such as recording electrodes and transducers that may be used to monitor the activity of specific physiological processes in either a research or clinical setting. They encompass the many complexities of remote monitoring and telemetry and include the requirements of emergency vehicles, operating rooms, and intensive care units.

Biomedical engineering involves applying the concepts, knowledge, and approaches of virtually all engineering disciplines (e.g. electrical, mechanical, and chemical engineering) to solve specific health care related problems. Because human health is multifaceted—involving not only our physical bodies but also the things that we put in our bodies (such as foods, pharmaceuticals, and medical devices) and the things that we put on our bodies (such as protective clothing and contact lenses)—the opportunities for interaction between engineers and health care professionals are many and varied.

Biomedical Engineering is thus an interdisciplinary branch of engineering heavily based both in engineering and in the life sciences ranging from theoretical, nonexperimental undertakings to state-of-the-art applications. It can encompass research, development, implementation, and operation. Accordingly, like medical practice itself, it is unlikely that any single person can acquire expertise that encompasses the entire field.[2] As a result, there has been an explosion of biomedical engineering specialists to cover this broad spectrum of activity. Yet, because of the interdisciplinary nature of this activity, there is considerable interplay and overlapping of interest and effort between them. For example, biomedical engineers engaged in the development of biosensors may interact with those interested in prosthetic devices to develop a means to detect and use the same bioelectric signal to power a prosthetic device.[3] Those engaged in automating the clinical chemistry laboratory may collaborate with those developing expert systems to assist clinicians in making clinical decisions based on specific laboratory data.[4] The possibilities are endless.

◆ *Source: Introduction to Biomedical Engineering—What is Biomedical Engineering?*

Glossary

professional [prəˈfeʃənəl]	n. 专业人员
telemetry [təˈlɛmətri]	n. 遥测技术；遥感勘测
multifaceted [ˌmʌltiˈfæsɪtɪd]	adj. 多层面的
transducer [trænzˈdusə]	n. 传感器
pharmaceuticals [ˌfɑːməˈsjuːtɪkəlz]	n. 药物
interdisciplinary [ˌɪntəˌdɪsəˈplɪnəri]	adj. 跨学科的
biosensor [ˈbaɪoˌsɛnsə]	n. 生物传感器
power [ˈpaʊə]	vt. 使……运转

Technical Terms

biomedical engineering	生物医学工程
multiphasic screening facilities	多相筛检设施
recording electrode	记录电极
ambulance	急救车
operating room	手术室
intensive care units	重症监护病房
engineering discipline	工程学科
health care	医疗保健
protective clothing	防护服
contact lenses	隐形眼镜
state-of-the-art	最新式的
bioelectric signal	生物电信号
prosthetic device	假肢

Notes

1. Many of the problems health professionals confronting today are of extreme importance to the engineer because they involve the fundamental aspects of device and systems analysis, design, and practical application—all of which lie at the heart of processes that are fundamental to engineering practice.

今天，健康专业人士面对的很多问题对工程师来说都极其重要，因为这些问题涉及设备和系统的分析、设计与实际应用，而这又是工程实践基础程序的核心。

分析：which lie at the heart...为非限定性定语从句，修饰 the fundamental aspects of...。

2. Accordingly, like medical practice itself, it is unlikely that any single person can acquire expertise that encompasses the entire field.

因此，与医疗实践一样，任何一个人不可能获得包含整个领域的专业知识。

分析：that 引导限定性定语从句，修饰 expertise。

3. For example, biomedical engineers engaged in the development of biosensors may interact

with those interested in prosthetic devices to develop a means to detect and use the same bioelectric signal to power a prosthetic device.

例如，参与开发生物传感器的生物医学工程师们，可以与那些对假肢感兴趣的工程师们合作，共同开发能检测生物电信号并同时用该信号驱动的假肢。

分析：engaged 前省略连接词 that，engaged in the development 修饰 biomedical engineers。

4. Those engaged in automating the clinical chemistry laboratory may collaborate with those developing expert systems to assist clinicians in making clinical decisions based on specific laboratory data.

那些投身于建设自动化临床化学实验室的工程师们，与需要专业实验数据来开发专家系统（在临床诊断中评估患者）的工程师们可以相互合作。

Translation Skills：生物医学工程各个领域名称

Biomechanics	生物力学	Biosensors	生物传感器
Medical Imaging	医学影像	Biomaterials	生物材料
Biotechnology	生物技术	Bioinformatics	生物信息学
Neural Engineering	神经工程	Tissue Engineering	组织工程
Physiological Modeling	生理建模	Biomedical Instrumentation	生物医学仪器
Clinical Engineering	临床工程	Rehabilitation Engineering	康复工程
Prosthesis	假体	Bionanotechnology	生物纳米技术
Biomedical Optics	生物医学光学	Artificial Organ	人工器官
Genetic Engineering	基因工程	Pharmaceutical Engineering	制药工程

1.2　Listening: Biomedical Engineering

Section 1

①

Biomedical engineering (BME), also known as bioengineering, is the application of engineering principles and design concepts to medicine and biology for healthcare purposes (e.g. diagnostic or therapeutic). This field seeks to close the gap between engineering and medicine, combining the design and problem solving skills of engineering with medical biological sciences to advance health care treatment, including diagnosis, monitoring and therapy. Also included under the scope of a biomedical engineer is the management of current medical equipment within hospitals while adhering to relevant industry standards. This involves equipment recommendations, procurement, routine testing and preventative maintenance, through decommissioning and disposal. This role is also known as a Biomedical Equipment Technician (BMET) or clinical engineering.

Biomedical engineering has only recently emerged as a new study, as compared to many other engineering fields. Such an evolution is common as a new field transitions from being an

---

① 本书各个单元听力部分的音频可扫描二维码获取。

interdisciplinary specialization among already-established fields, to being considered a field in itself. Much of the work in biomedical engineering consists of research and development, spanning a broad array of subfields. Prominent biomedical engineering applications include the development of biocompatible prostheses, various diagnostic and therapeutic medical devices ranging from clinical equipment to micro-implants, common imaging equipment such as MRIs and EKG/ECGs, regenerative tissue growth, pharmaceutical drugs and therapeutic biologicals.

🎧 Section 2

Some of the subfields of biomedical engineering are:

- Bioinformatics. Bioinformatics is an interdisciplinary field that develops methods and software tools for understanding biological data. As an interdisciplinary field of science, bioinformatics combines computer science, statistics, mathematics and engineering to analyze and interpret biological data.
- Biomechanics. Biomechanics is the study of the structure and function of the mechanical aspects of biological systems, at any level from whole organisms to organs, cells and cell organelles, using the methods of mechanics.
- Biomaterials. A biomaterial is any matter, surface or construct that interacts with living systems.
- Biomedical optics. Biomedical optics refers to the interaction of biological tissue and light, and how this can be exploited for sensing, imaging and treatment.
- Tissue engineering. One of the goals of tissue engineering is to create artificial organs (via biological material) for patients that need organ transplants. Biomedical engineers are currently exploring methods of creating such organs. Researchers have grown solid jawbones and tracheas from human stem cells towards this end. Several artificial urinary bladders have been grown in laboratories and transplanted successfully into human patients. Bioartificial organs, which use both synthetic and biological component, are also a focus area in research, such as with hepatic assist devices that use liver cells within an artificial bioreactor construct.

🎧 Section 3

- Genetic engineering.
- Neural engineering.
- Pharmaceutical engineering. This is an extremely broad category—essentially covering all health care products that do not achieve their intended results through predominantly chemical (e.g. pharmaceuticals) or biological (e.g. vaccines) means, and do not involve metabolism.
- Medical devices.

    A medical device is intended for use in:

    ➢ the diagnosis of disease or other conditions, or

➤ in the cure, mitigation, treatment or prevention of disease.

Some examples include pacemakers, infusion pumps, the heart-lung machine, dialysis machines, artificial organs, implants, artificial limbs, corrective lenses, cochlear implants, ocular prosthetics, facial prosthetics, somato prosthetics and dental implants.

● Medical imaging.

● Implants.

● Bionics.

● Clinical engineering. Clinical engineering is the branch of biomedical engineering dealing with the actual implementation of medical equipment and technologies in hospitals or other clinical settings.

● Rehabilitation engineering. Rehabilitation engineering is the systematic application of engineering sciences to design, develop, adapt, test, evaluate, apply and distribute technological solutions to problems confronted by individuals with disabilities.

◆ *Source: https://en.wikipedia.org/wiki/Biomedical_engineering.*

Listening Exercises

Listen to each section twice, and as you are listening, (a) number the words or expressions in the list on the work sheet by order of their first appearance in the passage you are listening to; (b) check if your numbering is correct—if incorrect, listen to the section again; (c) orally answer the questions about the content of each section.

Unit 1, Section 1

bioengineering	monitoring	regenerative
decommissioning	procurement	spanning
interdisciplinary	prostheses	therapeutic

1. What is a diagnosis? Explain the term in your own words and give one concrete example of a diagnosis.

2. Give an example of a medical condition that needs to be monitored over a longer time period.

3. Name three tasks that need to be carried out by a biomedical equipment technician.

Unit 1, Section 2

bioartificial	hepatic	tracheas
bioinformatics	organelles	transplants
construct	sensing	via

1. What do you need to study and be good at for a specialization in bioinformatics?

2. What is an organelle?

3. What is needed for growing an artificial urinary bladder?

Unit 1, Section 3

category	dialysis	mitigation
confronted	implementation	predominantly
diagnosis	infusion	somato

1. What is the difference between cure and mitigation?

2. Where does a cochlear implant go?

3. When does a person need a dialysis machine?

1.3　Writing: Why Do You Have to Write

English Scientific Papers?

　　撰写科技论文的目的有很多种。例如，与其他学者分享新的研究结果，发现了新的研究问题，介绍自己的研究成果等。著名学者 Faraday 曾经写道："There are three necessary steps in useful research: the first to begin it, the second to end it, and the third to publish it." 此外，发表科技论文的目的也可能是为了职称晋升或者申请科研经费。研究生可能需要发表几篇论文才能毕业。论文的数量和质量是学生和导师事业发展的敲门砖。"不成文，便成仁"（publish or perish）是学术生涯的写照。

　　上述目的虽然都是很重要的动机，然而就撰写科技论文而言，首要的目的是一种更狭义、更具体的目的，即把某些信息传达给某个读者群。

　　因此，在撰写科技论文时应记住，能否准确清晰地将论文内容有效地传达给读者群，是作者的责任，而不是读者的责任。一个研究结果只有在被别人使用时才有意义。而想被别人使用，论文必须能引起其他科学家的兴趣，而且要保证其他人能看懂并可以重复和再现研究结果。只有可以被理解的研究才会被重复，也只有可以被再现的作品才能被关注和引用。而论文被引用的数量常常用来衡量研究的影响力。从某种角度看，写作就像是把工作成果推销给其他科学家。因此，加强沟通技巧，学习科技论文标准的写作风格，无疑是研究人员科研训练中很重要的一部分。唯有通过这方面的训练，科学家和工程师才能更有效地将报告内容传达给读者群，才能更好地达到撰写报告的基本目的，即"有效的沟通"。

　　撰写科技论文的同时也培养了研究人员严谨思考的习惯。研究人员需要学习科技论文写作的另一个理由是，只有论文写得清楚、简洁、准确，才能反映出作者严谨、清晰的思维。相应地，如果研究人员无法清楚地表达自己的想法，那么就表明研究人员的思路不够清晰。撰写科技论文时千万不要以为有很好的想法或实验结果是最重要的事情，从而忽略了准确、清晰、简洁的表达方式。事实上，如果研究人员不知道如何表达自己的想法或者觉得自己表达得不好，通常问题不是表达能力不足，而是思维还有些模糊和粗糙。此时应对论文的写作思路和主题思想做进一步的分析，然后使用清楚、准确的言辞来表达自己的想法。此外，由于思考和语言的使用之间具有密切的联系，因此训练自己写出思路更清晰、结构更严谨的论文，同时也培养了自己严谨思考的习惯。

如何写出好的英文科技论文

- 好的科技论文需要创新性。在已沉寂的研究领域提出新的思想，在十分活跃的研究领域取得重大的进展，或者将原来彼此无联系的研究领域融合在一起，都是论文创新性的表现。一篇科技论文一定要提供新的信息，新的信息包括新的学术思想、新的实验方法或者新的发现。

- 好的科技论文要做到可读性强。结构严谨、环环相扣、首尾呼应的论文可读性更强。同时论文要有充分的论证和通顺的行文逻辑，以合理的方式再现作者的思路，使读者最终能得出与作者相同的结论。论文的语言表达应做到深入浅出、言简意赅。专业术语使用准确且前后一致，图表使用要合理规范，恰到好处。

- 在撰写英文科技论文时，应尽量把每个句子的意思都表达清晰，避免造成读者的误解。一篇好论文能使读者（特别是编辑与审稿人）在最短时间内准确地掌握作者的研究工作中最重大的科学价值。作者要明确地传达论文的结论和相关信息，对重要观点直接表述，防止语义含糊使读者推测论文观点。小说的写作需要埋伏笔、隐藏线索，但是英文科技论文的写作需要清晰明确地引导读者追随你的逻辑与观点。

- 英文科技论文的写作应尽量简洁。当论文中有复杂的长句时，应将其改写为简短、直接的句子，同时删掉句子中可有可无的词语。

英文科技论文写作重要的三个原则——"the three Cs"

"the three Cs"是英文科技论文写作重要的原则，在撰写科技论文时，应谨记于心。

- 正确（Correct）：句子的语法必须正确，而且论文的内容也要正确。
- 清楚（Clear）：作者的意图要表达清楚并且准确，使读者能够迅速读懂。
- 简洁（Concise）：论文的语言应简洁、明了，避免重复和冗长。每个句子中的每个单词都应是句子不可或缺的部分。

1.4　Speaking: English Conference Presentation

科研人员常常需要参加国际学术会议（international conference）或讨论会（seminar），并以做报告的方式讲解自己最近的研究成果。此外，各领域中的专业人员，如工业界的工程师与经理常常需要和同事开会，介绍研发计划、技术报告、市场分析报告或新产品数据等。本节将讨论如何准备英语会议报告，以及如何在会议中陈述自己的报告。

表示会议的单词

会议的英语表达方式有很多，包括 meeting、conference、congress、symposium、seminar、workshop、forum 等，这些词语的区别如下。

- Meeting：会议，最一般的用词，规模可大可小，层次可高可低。可以是正式或者是非正式的聚会，如首脑会议、紧急会议、告别会议等。
- Conference：大会，较为正式的用词，使用范围较广泛，多数国际会议使用该词语，如 International Conference on Biomedical Engineering。

- Congress：代表大会，由正式代表出席的会议，一般规模较大，如国际生物医学代表大会、全国人民代表大会（The National People's Congress）。
- Symposium：研讨会，主要指专题性的学术会议，尤其是参与者既为听众，又为报告人的会议。研讨会通常范围较窄，主题较突出，如 International Symposium on Biomaterials。
- Seminar：讨论会、组会，包括教授定期与学生讨论研究报告和发现的组会、研究生的专题讨论会，如 research seminar 等。
- Workshop：经验交流会、讨论会，强调信息（包括知识和经验）通常在较少的参与者之间的交流与交换，强调实际操作，如 workshop on gait analysis（步态分析经验交流会）。
- Forum：论坛、公众会议、讨论大众关心问题的集会，如 World Economic Forum （世界经济论坛）。

Unit 2　Genomics and Bioinformatics

2.1　Text: Genomics and Bioinformatics

Bioinformatics represents a new field at the interface of the ongoing revolutions in molecular biology and computers. Bioinformatics is defined as the use of computer databases and computer algorithms to analyze proteins, genes, and the complete collection of deoxyribonucleic acid (DNA) that comprises an organism (the genome). A major challenge in biology is to make sense of the enormous quantities of sequence data and structural data that are generated by genome-sequencing projects, proteomics, and other large-scale molecular biology efforts.[1] The tools of bioinformatics include computer programs that help to reveal fundamental mechanisms underlying biological problems related to the structure and function of macromolecules, biochemical pathways, disease processes, and evolution.[2]

While the discipline of bioinformatics focuses on the analysis of molecular sequences, genomics and functional genomics are two closely related disciplines. The goal of genomics is to determine and analyze the complete DNA sequence of an organism, that is, its genome. The DNA encoding genes can be expressed as ribonucleic acid (RNA) transcripts and then, in many cases, further translated into protein. Functional genomics describes the use of genome-wide assays to study gene and protein function. For humans and other species, it is now possible to characterize an individual's genome, collection of RNA (transcriptome), proteome and even the collections of metabolites and epigenetic changes, and the catalog of organisms inhabiting the body (the microbiome).

The fields of bioinformatics and genomics can be summarized with three perspectives. The first perspective on bioinformatics is the cell. Here we follow the central dogma. A focus of the field of bioinformatics is the collection of DNA (the genome), RNA (the transcriptome), and protein sequences (the proteome) that have been amassed. These millions-quadrillions of molecular sequences present both great opportunities and great challenges. A bioinformatics approach to molecular sequence data involves the application of computer algorithms and computer databases to molecular and cellular biology. Such an approach is sometimes referred to as functional genomics. This typifies the essential nature of bioinformatics: biological questions can be approached from levels ranging from single genes and proteins to cellular pathways and networks or even whole-genomic responses.[3]

From the cell we can focus on individual organisms, which represents a second perspective of the field of bioinformatics. Each organism changes across different stages of development and (for multicellular organisms) across different regions of the body. For example, while we may sometimes think of genes as static entities that specify features such as eye color or height, they are in fact dynamically regulated across time and region and in response to physiological state.[4]

At the largest scale is the tree of life. There are many millions of species alive today, and they can be grouped into the three major branches of bacteria, archaea, and eukaryotes. Molecular sequence databases currently hold DNA sequence from ~300,000 different species. The complete genome sequences of thousands of organisms are now available.

◆ *Source: Bioinformatics and Functional Genomics, 3rd edition.*

Glossary

bioinformatics [ˌbaɪəʊɪnfəˈmætɪks]	*n.* 生物信息学
genome [ˈdʒiːnəʊm]	*n.* 基因组
proteomics [ˌprəʊtɪˈɒmɪks]	*n.* 蛋白质组学
macromolecule [ˌmækrəˈmɒləkjʊl]	*n.* 大分子
transcriptome [trænˈskrɪptəʊm]	*n.* 转录组
proteome [ˈprəʊtɪəʊm]	*n.* 蛋白质组
metabolite [mɛˈtæbəˌlaɪt]	*n.* 代谢物
amass [əˈmæs]	*vt.* 积累
typify [ˈtɪpɪfaɪ]	*vt.* 代表
bacteria [bækˈtɪərɪə]	*n.* 细菌
archaea [ɑˈkiə]	*n.* 古生菌
eukaryotes [juˈkærɪəts]	*n.* 真核细胞

Technical Terms

molecular biology	分子生物学
computer database	计算机数据库
computer algorithm	计算机算法
deoxyribonucleic acid	脱氧核糖核酸
sequence data	序列数据
structural data	结构化数据
genome-sequencing projects	基因组测序计划
biochemical pathway	生化途径
disease process	疾病过程
molecular sequence	分子序列
genomics and functional genomics	基因组学和功能基因组学
ribonucleic acid (RNA) transcripts	核糖核酸（RNA）转录物
genome-wide assays	基因组广谱分析
epigenetic changes	表观遗传变异
central dogma	中心法则
millions-quadrillions	数以百万计
cellular biology	细胞生物学

Notes

1. A major challenge in biology is to make sense of the enormous quantities of sequence data and structural data that are generated by genome-sequencing projects, proteomics, and other large-scale molecular biology efforts.

生物学的一个主要挑战是理解在基因组测序计划、蛋白质组学和其他大规模分子生物学研究中产生的大量序列数据和结构数据。

分析： make sense of 意为"懂得，了解……的意义"。

2. The tools of bioinformatics include computer programs that help to reveal fundamental mechanisms underlying biological problems related to the structure and function of macromolecules, biochemical pathways, disease processes, and evolution.

生物信息学以计算机程序为工具，揭示与大分子的结构和功能、生化途径、疾病过程和进化等相关的生物学问题的基本机理。

分析： that 用作关系代词，引导限定性定语从句，先行词为 computer programs。

3. This typifies the essential nature of bioinformatics: biological questions can be approached from levels ranging from single genes and proteins to cellular pathways and networks or even whole-genomic responses.

这代表了生物信息学的本质特征：生物学问题可以从单一基因和蛋白质、细胞途径和网络甚至全基因组反应等不同的层面来探讨。

4. For example, while we may sometimes think of genes as static entities that specify features such as eye color or height, they are in fact dynamically regulated across time and region and in response to physiological state.

例如，有时我们会认为基因是确定诸如眼睛颜色或身高等特征的静态实体，但实际上它们是随时间和区域动态调整的，并能对生理状态做出响应。

分析： while 意为"虽然，尽管"，引导让步状语从句。

Translation Skills：专业英语的特点与翻译标准

随着全球化进程的加速，各国之间科技和学术交流也日益频繁。我们国家无论是在政治、经济，还是科学技术方面，在国际上所占的地位都越来越重要，近年来主持召开的国际性学术会议也越来越多。因此，生物医学工程专业领域的工作者必须具备良好的基础英语能力和专业英语能力，才能快速、准确、高效地吸收最新技术情报，参与国际科学技术交流，进而紧跟该专业领域的技术发展。

专业英语以其独特的语体，明确地表达作者在其专业方面的见解，表达方式直截了当，具有准确、精练、正式、逻辑性强的特点。专业英语属于科技英语的范畴，具有科技英语的特点，与专业内容联系紧密。通过专业英语的学习，研究人员不仅能掌握大量的专业词汇，还能熟悉专业英语的词法、句法的特点，从而提高专业英语的听、说、读、写能力。

专业英语的特点

相较于普通英语来说，专业英语的写作目的是准确地向读者传达科技概念、客观规律、理论和事实，所以更加注重叙述逻辑的缜密以及表达上的清晰与准确，较少使用晦涩或表露主观倾向和个人感情的词语。这些都决定了专业英语有其独特的语法特点、文体和表达风格。

（1）专业英语中多用动词的现在时，尤其是多用一般现在时来叙述事实或真理，客观地表述定义、定律、定理、方程式、公式、图表等。专业英语中用一般过去时来介绍实验情况或叙述事物的发展过程等，用一般将来时叙述计划要做的工作和预期获得的结果等。

例句

In the Biomedical Engineering field, many issues <u>exist</u> in the electronic medical devices repairing process, especially when the problem is intermittent.

在生物医学工程领域中，电子医疗设备的修复过程中<u>存在</u>着许多问题，尤其是间歇性问题。

This organizational structure <u>emphasizes</u> the integration and collaboration between a spectrum of technical expertise for clinical support and equipment management roles.

这种组织结构<u>强调</u>为临床支持提供一系列技术专业知识与设备管理角色之间的整合和协作。

（2）专业英语的专业性很强，专业术语、合成词及半技术词汇多。这些专业术语和词汇大都有着精确和单一的含义。即使是同一个词，由于学科和专业的不同，其含义往往也是不同的。

例句

The <u>connection</u> has come loose due to vibration.

震动使一些接线松了。

此处句中没有出现 wire 之类表示"线"的词，但专业知识使我们通过 connection 就很自然地想到"接线"或"连接线"。

We assume there are two variables in the <u>function</u>.

function 这个词，在大多数情况下指的是"功能"的意思，而如果出现在与数学或计算机语言相关的专业科技文献中多指"函数"的意思。

此外，更有一些术语和词汇已经在国际上形成了固定的范式，如生物医学工程里的"磁共振成像"（Magnetic Resonance Imaging，MRI），控制领域中的"频域分析法"（frequency domain analysis），经济学领域中的"马太效应"（Matthew effect），航空科技领域中的"空中交通信息服务"（Air Traffic Information Service，ATIS），等等。从上述例子中不难发现，由于范式的存在，科技英语词汇中会出现大量的缩略词，用来简单明了地表示某些具有固定意义的词汇。

从句子层面来说，专业英语多以客观陈述为主，且广泛使用被动语态。首先，科技论文陈述的是客观现象，介绍的是科技成果，所以使用被动句可以减少作者的主观色彩。其次，被动语态更能突出要论证、说明的对象，把它放在句子的主语位置上，就更能引人注目。而且在很多情况下，被动结构比主动结构更简单。

例句

<u>It is generally agreed that</u> 50% ~ 60% of the bone's mechanical competence can be explained by variations in the apparent density (bone mass/tissue volume).

人们普遍认为，50%～60%的骨骼机械能力可以通过表观密度（骨质量/组织体积）的变化来解释。

值得注意的是，it 是科技文献中一种客观表达的典范。

（3）专业英语多用结构复杂的长句。为了更好地体现要表达的原理、逻辑关系等，必须借助于层次分明、重点突出的复合长句。科学思维的复杂性也因而体现在专业英语的长句特征上。有时一个长句就是一个较长的段落。

例句

The method's performance has been evaluated in terms of its sensitivity to resolution and image rotation and the characteristic differences between TB anisotropy computed from transverse and longitudinal sections have been examined.

我们已经从该方法对分辨率和图像旋转的敏感度两方面对其进行了评估，并且已经检查了从横向和纵向截面计算的 TB 各向异性之间的特征差异。

Many accident victims are rushed to emergency rooms for treatment, and actions performed in the first few minutes after arrival can often mean the difference between life and death. Emergency room treatment has improved enormously over the past few decades, chiefly due to advances in the technology for looking inside of people quickly and accurately.

许多事故受害者被紧急送往急诊室接受治疗。而在他们到达急诊室后的几分钟内，医生采取的行动往往是生死攸关的。在过去的几十年中，急诊室治疗得到了极大的改善，主要是由于技术的进步，使得医生可以快速而准确地检查患者的身体。

（4）专业英语多使用虚拟语气。由于科技论文中的很多内容都是有关科学家们对事物和现象的论证及探索，因此常常涉及各种条件，所以使用虚拟语气的句子较多。此外，科研人员在表达他们对各种问题的看法时，为了使口气委婉，也常常使用虚拟语气。

例句

It would then appear that a better compromise could have been achieved. In a frictionless machine, the inequality of the above equation would become an equality.

这样看来，一种更好的妥协可能已经实现。在摩擦为零的机器中，上述不等式将变为等式。

（5）专业英语多使用祈使句。由于科技论文的一个重要特点就是所述理论的可解释性、所做实验的可重复性，因此，语句没有必要指明主语。命题、解题、顺序论证、实验指导、操作说明、工艺介绍、文献注释等多用祈使句。

例句

Now let K equal to zero, then we obtain the following equation.

让 K 等于零，则会得到下列等式。

（6）为了达到明确和简练的要求，在专业英语中多采用名词和介词短语。

例句

In this article, we present fundamental properties of topological structure of a 3D digitized picture, and provide a method to treat topology of digitized 3D figure.

本文给出了<u>三维数字化图形拓扑结构</u>的基本性质，并给出了一种处理三维数字化图形拓扑结构的方法。

Changes resulting from this evaluation may be the only way to assure and maintain <u>leadership and recognition from the BME community</u>.

评估结果的变化可能是确保和保持 <u>BME</u> 社区的领导和认可的唯一途径。

翻译标准

我国著名思想家、翻译家严复在其译作《天演论》中提出了翻译的三大准则"信、达、雅"。"信"指忠实、不悖原文，译文要做到客观准确，不偏离，不遗漏，也不要随意更改原文所要表达的意思；"达"指译文应通顺达意，避免刻意追求遵循原文形式，而使译文晦涩不通；"雅"指的是在"信""达"的基础上，译文要优美自然，追求译文本身的文采修辞。

严复提出的这三大准则，是翻译活动普遍遵循的规律，对各种英语文体的翻译都具有指导意义，也同样适用于专业英语的翻译。但是由于专业英语相较于其他类英语论文而言，有其独特的成文特点，所以在"信、达、雅"三原则落实到专业英语的翻译中时，也就被赋予了独特的内涵。

专业英语的翻译应遵循以下规律。

（1）**准备充分，有的放矢。**翻译专业英语时，译者除了要具备良好的英语素养，把握住翻译的一般规律，还要有相关专业和领域的知识储备。科技文献往往专业性很强，使用大量的专业术语和词汇。而且随着科技日新月异的发展，专业术语和词汇不断增多，相关的理论研究也不断丰富。所以在进行专业英语的翻译之前，做好相关的知识储备是很有必要的。

例句

Under Medicare, each <u>CPT</u> and <u>HCPCS II code</u> is assigned to an <u>Ambulatory Payment Classification (APC)</u> group with a unique relative weight, which is then converted into a payment amount.

在医保中，每个 <u>CPT</u> 和 <u>HCPCS II</u> 码均被分配到<u>门诊支付分类（APC）</u>组并具有唯一的相对权重，然后将其转换为付款金额。

这句话中有许多专业词汇和缩略词，需要译者对医疗场景及其相关的背景知识有一定的了解。

（2）**准确严谨。**与普通英语相比，专业英语的翻译对忠于原文的要求更高。科技文献在写作时更加强调逻辑严谨，表述准确。我们在翻译时也应少用或不用描述性形容词以及具有抒情作用的副词、感叹词及疑问词，并恰当地使用科技词汇、专业技术用语；同时译者应尊重客观事实，不回避不易翻译的语句，更不能随意改动数据，或加进自己的主观想象，进行自由翻译。此外，专业英语的翻译不应晦涩难懂，其准确性不能只停留在表层意义和文本形式的表达，而应该是在把握内涵和深层意义后将其准确传达。

例句

On account of the accuracy and ease with which resistance measurements may be made and the well-known manner in which resistance varies with temperature, <u>it is common to</u> use this variation to indicate changes in temperature.

由于电阻的大小是随温度的变化而变化的，而且用电阻进行测量既精确又方便。因此，电阻的变化通常用来指示温度的变化。

句子的主体结构是 it is common to，介词短语 on account of 作原因状语，第二个 and 作为连接 accuracy and ease 和 well-known manner 的并列连词。要翻译这样的长句，译者需要厘清头绪，对原句结构进行重组，改变原来的语序。

（3）顺畅通达。译文的表达应该自然连贯、通俗易懂，要符合现代汉语的用语规范，避免死译和硬译、结构混乱、逻辑不清等现象。这就要求译者在理解原文内容的基础上，用汉语恰如其分地将作者的意图表述出来。要使译文表达得通顺，最重要的一点是规范造句。在遵循正确的语法规则、语言习惯及修辞艺术的基础上去组织译文的句子。同时，要重视语序的安排，时态、语态的表达，虚词的恰当使用，复合句结构的安排等。此外，要特别注意专业英语中的语言结构，如后置定语、名词化结构、被动语态、非限定性动词等。在具体翻译时要灵活处理，合理翻译。

例句

Railways are the top mode of transportation for most Chinese passengers. National conditions including a great population and a low average personal income are reasons for this.

原句：铁路是我国大部分旅客首选的交通方式。我国人口众多和人均收入相对较低的现实国情是造成这种状况的原因。

英语原文将原因放在后面，但根据汉语"原因在前，结果在后"的逻辑思维习惯，翻译时最好将原因提前。调整语序后，信息会更加明确，语句也更为连贯。

修改后：我国人口众多和人均收入相对较低的现实国情，决定了铁路是我国大部分旅客首选的交通方式。

（4）客观科学。科技文献是对科学事实和科学理论进行的客观描述和阐释，而严格规范的语句和措辞是保证译文科学性的前提。为确保译文的科学性，应重视专业术语的翻译。专业术语是科技文献的重要组成部分，是科学理论的语言基础，也是各领域、各专业特色的代表。除了大量国际统一的专业术语，译者还应在忠于原文的基础上，力求用最科学的语言进行表述。

例句

The 4K is essentially the resolution of 35mm film negative, but even when scanning second or third generation elements, we still start with a 4K scan.

原句：4K 解决的基本上是 35mm 的底片，或是第二代或第三代扫描的器件，我们用的是 4K 的扫描仪。

上述译文有两个根本性的错误，导致读者完全无法理解。一个是将 resolution 误译为"解决"，另一个是将 elements 误译为"器件"。第二个错误尤其离谱，因为扫描的对象从胶片变成了器件。

修改后：4K 基本上是 35mm 底片的分辨率，但即便是扫描第二代或第三代胶片，我们仍然采用 4K 扫描。

2.2　Listening: Genomics and Bioinformatics

 Section 1

Bioinformatics is an interdisciplinary field that develops methods and software tools for understanding biological data. As an interdisciplinary field of science, bioinformatics combines biology, computer science, mathematics and statistics to analyze and interpret biological data. Bioinformatics has been used for in silico analyses of biological queries using mathematical and statistical techniques.

Bioinformatics is both an umbrella term for the body of biological studies that use computer programming as part of their methodology, as well as a reference to specific analysis "pipelines" that are repeatedly used, particularly in the field of genomics. Common uses of bioinformatics include the identification of candidate genes and single nucleotide polymorphisms (SNPs). Often, such identification is made with the aim of better understanding the genetic basis of disease, unique adaptations, desirable properties (esp. in agricultural species), or differences between populations. In a less formal way, bioinformatics also tries to understand the organizational principles within nucleic acid and protein sequences, called proteomics.

 Section 2

Bioinformatics has become an important part of many areas of biology. In experimental molecular biology, bioinformatics techniques such as image and signal processing allow extraction of useful results from large amounts of raw data. In the field of genetics and genomics, it aids in sequencing and annotating genomes and their observed mutations. It plays a role in the text mining of biological literature and the development of biological and gene ontologies to organize and query biological data. It also plays a role in the analysis of gene and protein expression and regulation. Bioinformatics tools aid in the comparison of genetic and genomic data and more generally in the understanding of evolutionary aspects of molecular biology. At a more integrative level, it helps analyze and catalogue the biological pathways and networks which constitute an important part of systems biology. In structural biology, it aids in the simulation and modeling of DNA, RNA, proteins as well as biomolecular interactions.

 Section 3

To study how normal cellular activities are altered in different disease states, the biological data must be combined to form a comprehensive picture of these activities. Therefore, the field of bioinformatics has evolved such that the most pressing task now involves the analysis and interpretation of various types of data. This includes nucleotide and amino acid sequences, protein domains, and protein structures. The actual process of analyzing and interpreting data is referred to as computational biology. Important subdisciplines within bioinformatics and computational biology include:

- Development and implementation of computer programs that enable efficient access to, use and management of, various types of information.
- Development of new algorithms (mathematical formulas) and statistical measures that assess relationships among members of large data sets. For example, there are methods to locate a gene within a sequence, to predict protein structure and/or function, and to cluster protein sequences into families of related sequences.

The primary goal of bioinformatics is to increase the understanding of biological processes. What sets it apart from other approaches, however, is its focus on developing and applying computationally intensive techniques to achieve this goal. Examples include: pattern recognition, data mining, machine learning algorithms, and visualization. Major research efforts in the field include sequence alignment, gene finding, genome assembly, drug design, drug discovery, protein structure alignment, protein structure prediction, prediction of gene expression and protein-protein interactions, genome-wide association studies, the modeling of evolution and cell division/mitosis.

Listening Exercises

Listen to each section twice, and as you are listening, (a) number the words or expressions in the list on the work sheet by order of their first appearance in the passage you are listening to; (b) check if your numbering is correct—if incorrect, listen to the section again; (c) orally answer the questions about the content of each section.

Unit 2, Section 1

interdisciplinary	nucleotide	queries
interpret	organizational	repeatedly
methodology	proteomics	silico

1. What does a bioinformatician need to be good at for analyzing and interpreting biological data?

2. What is the purpose of studying nucleotide polymorphisms?

3. What is an "analysis pipeline"?

Unit 2, Section 2

analysis	catalogue	extraction
annotating	evolutionary	ontologies
biomolecular	expression	techniques

Unit 2, Section 3

algorithms	computationally	mitosis
cluster	implementation	pressing
computational	locate	states

1. How can one monitor altered cellular activities that indicate different disease states?

2. How can one locate a gene within a sequence, predict protein structure and functions?

3. How does bioinformatics differ from other approaches in its goal to increase the understanding of biological processes?

2.3　Writing: Sentence

英语句子的语序

英语有严格的语序，例如，"The authors posted their draft to the scientific journal."。
大多数的句子采用这种语序。该例句的主要句子成分包括：

- 主语（the authors）；
- 谓语动词（posted）；
- 直接宾语（their draft）；
- 间接宾语（the scientific journal）。

此外，句子成分还可能包括状语和补语等。保证语法正确的关键是保持句子的主干，即主语、谓语动词与宾语尽可能地靠近。

例句

Last Monday <u>the authors posted their draft to the scientific journal</u> for peer review.（正确）
<u>The authors</u> last Monday <u>posted</u> for peer review <u>their draft to the scientific journal</u>.（错误）

平时注意从教科书与科技论文中总结典型英语句式的语序，并与汉语的语序进行比较和分析，这样可以极大地提高英语的写作能力。

句式简洁原则

在科技论文的写作中，尽可能选择可以使句子更简洁的句式。试比较下列两个句式。

例句

句式 1：The physiological characteristics of the subjects <u>are shown</u> in Table 1.
句式 2：Table 1 <u>shows</u> the physiological characteristics of the subjects.

在科技论文中，经常可以看到这两种句式。主动语态使句式更简短，因此句式 2 的表述更好。

主语位于动词之前

在专业英语中，主语应出现在动词之前。

例句

In the present study participated <u>fifty subjects</u>.（错误）
<u>Fifty subjects</u> participated in the present study.（正确）

在开始描述之前，首先应该指明主语，即使目的是为了铺垫引出主语。

🎋例句

原句：Among the factors that influence the choice of parameters are <u>time and cost</u>.

修改后：<u>Time and cost</u> are among the factors that influence the choice of parameters.

主语与动词尽可能靠近

动词在句子中包含重要的信息。如上文提到的，英语句子中的主语与动词应尽可能地靠近。

🎋例句

原句：People with a high rate of intelligence, an unusual ability to resolve problems, a passion for computers, along with good communication skills <u>are generally employed by such companies.</u>

这个句子中动词出现得过晚，使重要的信息不能及时表达。

修改后：<u>Such companies generally employ people</u> with a high rate of intelligence, an unusual ability to resolve problems, a passion for computers, along with good communication skills.

修改后句子变为主动语态。在有些情况下可能需要使用被动语态，或者多个主语需要公用一个动词。在这种情况下，第一个主语后用被动语态。

<u>People with a high rate of intelligence are generally employed</u> by such companies. They must also have other skills including an unusual ability to resolve problems, a passion for computers, along with good communication skills.

避免在主语和动词之间插入附加说明

在主语和动词之间插入几个单词往往会干扰读者的思路，而且读者会认为插入的信息并不重要。简单易懂的句子往往逻辑通顺，语义连贯。

🎋例句

原句：<u>The result</u>, after the calculation has been made, <u>can be used to determine Y</u>.

修改后：After the calculation has been made, <u>the result can be used to determine Y</u>.

根据时间顺序，原句主语与动词之间插入的信息作为状语从句，位于句首。修改后使主语与动词连接构成完整的句子。

🎋例句

原句：<u>These steps</u>, owing to the difficulties in measuring the weight, <u>require some simplifications</u>.

修改后：Owing to the difficulties in measuring the weight, <u>these steps require some simplifications</u>.

或者：<u>These steps require some simplifications</u>, owing to the difficulties in measuring the weight.

修改后使主语与动词构成一个完整句子。附加信息作为从句位于句首还是句末，取决于从句的重要性。如果从句包含重要信息，可置于句首。

副词的位置

一般而言，副词的使用规则并不复杂。主要有以下 3 条。

（1）副词位于句中主要动词的前面。

Dying neurons do not <u>usually</u> exhibit these biochemical changes.

The mental functions are slowed, and patients are <u>often</u> confused.

（2）如果有两个助动词，副词位于句中第二个助动词的前面。

Late complications may not <u>always</u> <u>have</u> been notified.

（3）副词位于 be 动词的一般现在时或一般过去时之后。

The answer of the machine <u>is</u> <u>always</u> correct.

如果需要特别强调，一些副词（sometimes，occasionally，normally，usually）可以位于句首。

<u>Normally</u> X is used to do Y, but <u>occasionally</u> it can be used to do Z.

其他可以位于句首的词或短语包括：

- firstly，secondly，finally（列举）；
- moreover（对负面概念的进一步负面的支持）；
- since，although，despite the fact（表明一种让步或者开始进一步解释）；
- alternatively（表明另一种可能性）；
- surprisingly，intriguingly，regrettably，unfortunately（吸引注意力或者表达某种情感）；
- specifically，in particular（特指）。

避免创造一串名词用于描述一个概念

不能将没有内在联系的一串名词放在一起。例如，mass destruction weapons 的表述是不正确的，正确的表述为：weapons of mass destruction。

名词的叠加用法没有明确的规则，是一种习惯用法，是约定俗成的。在使用名词叠加用法时，最好用 Google Scholar 来确认这种用法是否已经存在，否则以英语为母语的审稿人会不认可这种用法。如果经过查找没有发现所使用的名词叠加用法，那么需要在名词之间添加介词。

小结

- 基本的英语语序：主语+谓语动词+直接宾语+间接宾语。无论有什么样的修饰，请保持这种语序，并使这几个主要成分尽量靠近。
- 如果有几个主语可选，尽量选择最相关、句式最短的主语。
- 主语不要出现得太晚，要尽量避免句子以 It 开头。
- 尽量避免在主语和动词之间插入附加说明。
- 大部分副词位于主要动词之前。
- 形容词位于所修饰的名词之前，不要在两个名词之间插入形容词。
- 不要毫无语感地将一串名词串联使用。

2.4　Speaking: Conference Presentation—Preparation

会议报告成功与否，在于报告人能否实施三个基本步骤：细致的准备（prepare thoroughly），勤奋的练习（practice diligently）以及有效的演讲（present effectively）。在英文中，这三个步骤称为"the three Ps"。

即使英文水平较高，报告人也仍然需要认真准备。Always OVERPREPARE！报告的目的是将信息传达给听众，因此需要尽量确保听众能够准确地理解报告的主要内容。另外，如果准备得充分，在做报告时就会缓解紧张情绪，把报告的内容有效地传达给听众。

Know Your Audience（了解听众）

（1）Who will I be speaking to?（我的报告讲给谁听？）

（2）What do they know about my topic already?（听众对我的报告主题了解多少？）

（3）What will they want to know about my topic?（听众期望从这个主题中了解什么内容？）

（4）What do I want them to know by the end of my talk?（报告结束后我希望听众能够记住什么？）

Main Points（重点）

在报告结束之后，听众会记得少数比较突显的内容。所以，不需要提供过多不必要的细节，而应选择几个重点，并尽量把这些重点表达清楚。

例如，在介绍自己的研究工作时，至少要将以下四个方面的重要内容表达清楚：

- Why we did this?（研究目的或动机）
- How we did it?（研究方法）
- What are the results?（研究结果）
- What does that mean?（研究结果的意义）

这四个方面和一般科技论文的组织结构（即引言、方法、结果、讨论）是相对应的。然而，会议报告的内容并不会像书面的研究报告一样详细。例如，在科技论文中，方法一章的目的在于详细描述作者的实验方法，以便让读者能重复作者的实验以确定其研究结果是否有效。相较之下，在会议报告中，我们并没有时间详细解释实验方法的所有细节。在简短的会议报告中，听众会暂时假设我们的实验方法没有重大的缺陷，所以只要简略地描述实验方法即可。对于如何描述研究结果这一问题，也需要应用相同的原则。无须列出所有数据，只要提供足够的数据以支持自己的结论即可。切勿提供过多的数据或复杂的表格，以免听众无法理解或根本看不出主要结果是什么。

Framework and Transitions（报告的框架和上下文的过渡）

选择报告的组织形式与框架，并以此来组织报告的内容和相关的资料。例如，如果需要介绍实验研究项目的结果，那么可以遵循论文的组织形式，即先解释研究背景及目的，再描述实验方法并列出研究结果，最后对结果的意义进行讨论。如果需要描述如何做某件事情或制造某种东西，则可以按照制造的步骤来组织报告的内容。如果需要比较两种不同的方法或技术，则可以采用比较与对照的组织形式。另外，要注意报告过程中的前后呼应和幻灯片之间的过渡。

Visual Aids（准备有效的视觉辅助）

视觉辅助（如图片、动图、视频等）是成功的会议报告不可或缺的部分。视觉辅助有几种重要的功能。

■ 视觉辅助能使听众的注意力集中在报告人所表达的内容上。当报告人需要强调某个重点时，最好能利用图片、视频等来表达，这样听众就会更容易记住重点内容。

■ 视觉辅助能帮助报告人清楚地、有效地将很复杂的信息传达给听众。有些信息难以用语言表达，而且仅以语言表达也常会令听众觉得迷惑。以图片等视觉辅助来表达会更清晰，效果会更好，一张图胜过千言万语（a picture is worth a thousand words）。例如，假设我们在科技报告中需要描述某种电子线路，利用图形以解释线路的结构一定比直接用语言描述容易得多。而且对听众而言，这样也更容易了解线路的结构。

Interesting Opening（引人入胜的开场）

最好设计一个良好的开场，引发听众的兴趣。在开场介绍中提供足够的背景资料，使听众了解报告的内容。可以一开始就明确表达自己的主要论点，以便听众知道报告将要提出哪些主要内容，在听报告的过程中，跟随报告人的思路。

Effective Summary（高效的总结）

在报告结束前，应以精简的方式强调重点——即最重要的结论或建议。再次有效地强调自己的主要论点，听众更容易对这些论点留下深刻的印象。

在有些情况下，叙述完结论还可以鼓励听众提出问题。

■ If there are any questions, I'd be happy to take them now.

■ If there are any questions, I'd be happy to answer them.

如果没有时间让听众提问，那么在做完总结之后，以"Thank you!"或"This concludes my report. Thank you!"结束报告。

Unit 3   Anatomy and Physiology

3.1   Text: Anatomy and Physiology

Human anatomy is the scientific study of the body's structures. Some of these structures are very small and can only be observed and analyzed with the assistance of a microscope. Other larger structures can readily be seen, manipulated, measured, and weighed. The word "anatomy" comes from a Greek root that means "to cut apart". Human anatomy was first studied by observing the exterior of the body and observing the wounds of soldiers and other injuries. Later, physicians were allowed to dissect bodies of the dead to augment their knowledge. When a body is dissected, its structures are cut apart in order to observe their physical attributes and their relationships to one another. Dissection is still used in medical schools, anatomy courses, and in pathology labs. In order to observe structures in living people, however, a number of imaging techniques have been developed. These techniques allow clinicians to visualize structures inside the living body such as a cancerous tumor or a fractured bone.

Anatomists take two general approaches to the study of the body's structures: regional and systemic. Regional anatomy is the study of the interrelationships of all of the structures in a specific body region, such as the abdomen. Studying regional anatomy helps us appreciate the interrelationships of body structures, such as how muscles, nerves, blood vessels, and other structures work together to serve a particular body region. In contrast, systemic anatomy is the study of the structures that make up a discrete body system—that is, a group of structures that work together to perform a unique body function.[1] For example, a systemic anatomical study of the muscular system would consider all of the skeletal muscles of the body.

Whereas anatomy is about structure, physiology is about function. Human physiology is the scientific study of the chemistry and physics of the structures of the body and the ways in which they work together to support the functions of life. Much of the study of physiology centers on the body's tendency toward homeostasis. Homeostasis is the state of steady internal conditions maintained by living things. The study of physiology certainly includes observation, both with the naked eye and with microscopes, as well as manipulations and measurements. However, current advances in physiology usually depend on carefully designed laboratory experiments that reveal the functions of the many structures and chemical compounds that make up the human body.[2]

Like anatomists, physiologists typically specialize in a particular branch of physiology. For example, neurophysiology is the study of the brain, spinal cord, and nerves and how these work together to perform functions as complex and diverse as vision, movement, and thinking.[3] Physiologists may work from the organ level (exploring, for example, what different parts of the brain do) to the molecular level (such as exploring how an electrochemical signal travels along nerves).

Form is closely related to function in all living things. For example, the thin flap of your eyelid can snap down to clear away dust particles and almost instantaneously slide back up to allow you to see again.[4] At the microscopic level, the arrangement and function of the nerves and muscles that serve the eyelid allow for its quick action and retreat. At a smaller level of analysis, the function of these nerves and muscles likewise relies on the interactions of specific molecules and ions. Even the three-dimensional structure of certain molecules is essential to their function.

◆ *Source: Anatomy and Physiology.*

Glossary

anatomy [ə'nætəmɪ]	*n.* 解剖学
dissect [dɪˌsekt]	*vt.* 解剖
pathology [pə'θɒlədʒi]	*n.* 病理（学）
anatomist [ə'nætəmɪst]	*n.* 解剖学家
homeostasis [ˌhomɪə'stesɪs]	*n.* 体内平衡
neurophysiology [ˌnʊrofɪzɪ'ɒlədʒi]	*n.* 神经生理学
eyelid ['aɪlɪd]	*n.* 眼睑，眼皮
ion ['aɪən]	*n.* 离子

Technical Terms

cancerous tumor	癌性肿瘤
regional anatomy	部位解剖学
skeletal muscles	骨骼肌
human physiology	人体生理学
center on	以……为中心
spinal cord	脊髓
electrochemical signal	电化学信号
thin flap	薄皮瓣

Notes

1. In contrast, systemic anatomy is the study of the structures that make up a discrete body system—that is, a group of structures that work together to perform a unique body function.

相比之下，全身解剖学研究的是构成独立身体系统的结构——即一组结构共同作用以执行特定身体功能。

分析："—"后接同位语，对 the structures that...进行补充说明。

2. However, current advances in physiology usually depend on carefully designed laboratory experiments that reveal the functions of the many structures and chemical compounds that make up the human body.

然而，目前生理学的进步通常依赖于精心设计的实验，以揭示构成人体的诸多结构和化合物的功能。

分析：句中出现两个 that，均引导限定性定语从句。

3. For example, neurophysiology is the study of the brain, spinal cord, and nerves and how these work together to perform functions as complex and diverse as vision, movement, and thinking.

例如，神经生理学研究大脑、脊髓和神经，以及它们如何协同工作以发挥视觉、运动和思维等复杂多样的功能。

分析：how these work…是由连词 how 引导的名词性从句。

4. For example, the thin flap of your eyelid can snap down to clear away dust particles and almost instantaneously slide back up to allow you to see again.

例如，眼睑的薄皮瓣可以向下闭合以清除粉尘，然后几乎瞬间向上滑回，让你能够再次视物。

分析：snap down 意为"推下，向下放"。

Translation Skills：专业英语构词法

专业英语中包含大量专业词汇和半专业词汇。专业词汇是指仅用于某一学科或专业的词汇或术语；半专业词汇是指各学科通用的词汇或术语。如果不懂得某一领域的专业术语或词汇，就不可能正确阅读和理解该领域的专业技术文献。专业词汇主要有以下几个特点：

■ 从古希腊语和拉丁语中吸收而来；
■ 词汇表述的意义精确且单一；
■ 通过使用前缀和后缀构成新词；
■ 词汇中大量出现缩略词。

在阅读专业技术文献和资料时，结合构词法中的构词理论可以有效地解决在专业英语翻译中的问题。专业英语中常见的构词法有以下几种。

1．词缀派生法

在专业英语中，常常在词根前、后分别加上前缀或后缀构成新词。

例句

However, regulatory issues are so deeply embedded into product design and development that innovators need to understand regulatory processes and nomenclature in order to provide effective leadership in the biodesign innovation process.

然而，监管问题深入产品设计和开发的方方面面。创新者们为了在生物设计创新过程中有效地起到领导作用，就需要了解监管程序和术语。

通常来说，在构成新词的过程中，加前缀构成的新词只改变词义，词的属性一般不会改变。下面列举一些常用前缀。

（1）anti-/counter-　表示"反，抗"

anti-interference　抗干扰；counterflow　反向流动；anti-radar　反雷达

（2）auto-　表示"自动，自"

autocontrol　自控；automoduation　自调制；automobile　自动车

（3）de-　表示相反动作

modulator　调制器　→　demodulator　解调器

（4）deci-　表示"十分之一"，常译为"分"

decibel（dB）　分贝；decimeter（dm）　分米；decigram（dg）　分克

（5）di-　表示"二"

dioxide　二氧化物；diode　二极管；dipole　偶极子

（6）dis-　对应单词的反义词

connect　连接　→　disconnect　解开；place　放置　→　displace　位移

close　关　→　disclose　揭露；trust　信任　→　distrust　怀疑

（7）in-　表示否定

accurate　精确的　→　inaccurate　不精确的；variable　可变的　→　invariable　不变的

visible　看得见的　→　invisible　看不见的；justice　公平　→　injustice　不公平

（8）inter-　表示"互相，（在）内，（在）中间"

interconnect　互连；interface　界面；interchange　互换

（9）micro-　表示"微，百万分之一"

microwave　微波；microfilm　微缩胶卷；microelectronic　微电子学

（10）mini-　表示"小"

minicell　微细胞；minicomputer　微型计算机；minibus　微型公共汽车

（11）over-　表示"超过，太"

overweight　超重；overfrequency　超频；overcharge　过量充电

（12）photo-　表示"光，光电，光敏"

photocell　光电池；photohead　光电传感头；photorectifier　光电检波器

（13）pre-　表示"在前，预先"

preheat　预热；preamplifier　前置放大器；pre-breakdown　未击穿前的

（14）re-　表示"再，重新"

produce　生产　→　reproduce　再生产；combine　结合　→　recombine　重新结合

（15）sub-　表示"下，低，亚，次，副"

sublinear　亚线性的；subcircuit　支路；subcode　子码

（16）tele-　表示"远"

television　电视；telescope　望远镜；telecontrol　遥控

（17）tri-　表示"三"

triangle　三角形；tricycle　三轮车；tricar　三轮汽车

（18）thermo-　表示"热"

thermo-emf　热电（动）势；thermoelectric　热电的；thermo-fuse　热熔丝

（19）ultra-　表示"超"

ultra-high-frequency　超高频；ultraportable　极轻便的；ultrasonic　超声的

（20）un-　表示相反，"不，非，未"等

unloading　去载；unequal　不等的；undecided　未决定的

（21）bi-　表示"双，重"

bipolar relay　双极继电器；bilateral　两边的，双边的；bimetal　双金属材料

（22）co-　表示"共，同，一起，相互"

coaxial cable　同轴电缆；coexist　共存

（23）equi-　表示"同等，均"

equipartition　均分；equilibrium　均衡，平衡

（24）hydro-　表示"水，氧化"

hydrodynamic　水力的，水压的，流体动力学的；hydroelectric　水力发电的

（25）hyper-　表示"高，超，重，极度"

hypersonic　超高速的；hypertension　高血压

（26）mal-　表示"不，失"

malfunction　失灵，故障；malformation　畸形

（27）mega-　表示"兆，百万"

megawatt　兆瓦；megaton　百万吨级

（28）multi-　表示"多"

multi-frequency　多频率

（29）post-　表示"后"

postfault　故障后

（30）semi-　表示"半"

semiconductor　半导体

加后缀构成新词，主要改变词的属性。下面列举一些常用后缀。

（1）-ance/-ence（名词词尾）

existence　存在；capacitance　电容；resonance　谐振

（2）-ary（形容词词尾）

element　元素 → elementary　初步的；moment　时刻 → momentary　瞬息的

（3）-en（动词词尾）　一般是形容词+en，表示"使……"

wide　宽的 → widen　加宽；soft　软 → soften　软化；short　短的 → shorten　缩短

（4）-fold　接在数词后，构成形容词或副词，表示"……倍"

three-fold　三倍的（地）；a thousand-fold　一千倍的（地）

（5）-free（形容词词尾）　表示"无……的，免于……的"

oil-free　无油的；dust-free　无尘的；loss-free　无损耗的

（6）-ful（形容词词尾）

success　成功 → successful　成功的；power　能力 → powerful　强有力的

（7）-ics（名词词尾）　表示学科名称

physics　物理学；mathematics　数学；electronics　电子学

（8）-ity（名词词尾）　构成抽象名词

reliable　可靠的 → reliability　可靠性；impure　不纯的 → impurity　杂质

（9）-ive（形容词词尾）

conduct　传导 → conductive　导电的；act　行为，行动 → active　起作用的，活跃的

（10）-less（形容词词尾）　表示"无……"

limit　极限 → limitless　无限的；wire　导线 → wireless　无线的

（11）-ment（名词词尾）

displace　转移 → displacement　位移；equip　装备 → equipment　设备

（12）-proof（形容词词尾）　表示"防……的"

waterproof　防水的；fireproof　防火的；lightningproof　防雷的

（13）-tion/-sion（名词词尾）

induce　感应；induction　感应

operate　工作；operation　工作，运算

transmit　发射；transmission　传输，发射

（14）-able（形容词词尾）

count　计算 → countable　可数的；compare　比较 → comparable　可比较的

（15）-al（形容词词尾）

digit　数字 → digital　数字的；function　功能 → functional　功能的

（16）-er/-or　表示"机器，设备，物件"等

air-oil booster　气-液增压器；air compressor　空气压缩机

inductor　电感器；operator　操作员

transmitter　发射机；switcher　切换器

（17）-meter　表示"……表，……计"

speedmeter　速度计；ohmmeter　电阻表

（18）-ist, -ician（名词词尾）　表示"从事某方面工作的人，……家"

optics　光学 → opticist　光学家；mechanics　机械学 → mechanician　机械师

（19）-ology　表示"研究或科学"

lexicology　词汇学；morphology　形态学

（20）-dom　表示"身份，地位，状态"

freedom　自由；kingdom　王国；boredom　厌倦、无聊

2．合成法

合成法就是把两个以上的单词组合成一个复合词，在词形结构上有时使用连字符，有时不使用连字符。使用这种方法组合成的新词汇在拼写方法、发音方法和语义上都会有些变化。在科技英语中，由于学科不断交叉发展，产生了大量的复合词。

📖例句

Without <u>regulatory clearance</u> by the FDA (or the equivalent agency abroad) even the most innovative and important breakthrough in medical technology will never reach patients.

如果没有通过美国食品药品监督管理局（或国外同等机构）<u>监管批准</u>，即使最新、最重大突破的医疗技术也无法应用到患者身上。

例句

The new law provided for three classes of medical devices based on risk, each requiring a different level of regulatory scrutiny.

基于风险，新的法律将医疗设备分为三类，每一类有不同等级的监管要求。

其他复合词举例：

nerve agent	神经性毒剂
reaction mechanism	反应机理
carbon steel	碳钢
overestimate	高估
film goers	电影观众
furrow-keratitis	钩状角膜炎
group-specific	类属特异性的
common-ion effect	同离子效应
acid ionization constant	酸离解常数
standard electrode potential	标准电极电位
full-enclosed	全封闭的
face-to-face	面对面
feedback	反馈
lunch box	便携式计算机
aircraft carrier	航空母舰
smart weapon	灵巧武器

3. 转化法

转化法就是把一个词从一种词性转化成另一种词性，但不改变词形的构词法。例如，某些形容词可以转化成名词，很多动词可以转化成名词，很多名词可以转化成动词等。

slow（*adj.* 慢的）——slow（*v.* 放慢）

water（*n.* 水）——water（*v.* 浇水）

form（*n.* 形式）——form（*v.* 形成）

heat（*adj.* 热的）——heat（*v.* 加热）

power（*n.* 动力）——power（*v.* 提供动力）

knowledge（*n.* 知识）——knowledge（*v.* 了解，知道）

forward（*adv.* 向前）——forward（*v.* 推进）

flow（*v.* 流动）——flow（*n.* 流量）

许多专业词汇都是由一般生活词语转化而成的，例如，

carrier（*n.* 搬运工）——carrier（*n.* 载体，载波，航空母舰，病毒携带者，传体）

chain（*n.* 链条）——chain（*n.* 山脉，电路）

fence（*n.* 栅栏）——fence（*n.* 雷达警戒网，电子篱笆）

beach（*n.* 海滩）——beach（*vi.* 搁浅）

cat（*n.* 猫）——cat（*n.* 起锚滑车，无线电遥控靶机）

egg（*n.* 鸡蛋）——egg（*n.* 航空炸弹，地雷，卵形物）

在对词义进行选择时，不要忘记语言是随着社会的发展而不断发展的，不是静止不变的，词的含义亦是如此。如 bird 一词，原意为"鸟"。随着科技的发展，其含义进一步扩大，可指飞机、火箭、直升机、航天飞机、卫星等任何飞行器。sail 一词原意为"帆"，自潜水艇出现以后，增添了"潜艇指挥塔"的含义。由此可见，词义是随时间的变迁、社会的发展而变化的，不应只停留在其原意上。

4．缩略法

随着社会和科技的快速发展，专业英语中的新术语大量涌现。其中，对于一些由两个或两个以上单词组成的词组，可以采用只取词头字母的方法进行缩写。例如，

EST：English for Science and Technology 科技英语

CAD：Computer Aided Design 计算机辅助设计

SCR：Silicon Controlled Rectifier 可控硅整流器

BME：Biomedical Engineering 生物医学工程

CT：Computerized Tomography 计算机层析成像

对于一个单词，仅保留其部分字母。例如，

lab：laboratory 实验室

Corp：corporation 股份公司

Co.,Ltd.：Corporation Limited 股份有限公司

kg：kilogram 千克

m.p.：melting point 熔点

rpm（r/m）：revolution per minute 转/分钟

5．混成法

将两个单词分别取一部分组合在一起，从而构成一个新词。例如，

alcohol + dehydrogenation ⇒ aldehyde 醛、乙醛

medical ｜ care ⇒ medicare 医疗保健

positive + electron ⇒ positron 正电子

modulator + demodulator ⇒ modem 调制解调器

transfer + resistor ⇒ transistor 晶体管

6．借用法

英语在其发展的过程中吸收了很多外来词汇，如希腊语、拉丁语、法语、西班牙语、阿拉伯语等语言中的词汇。在这些语言中，希腊语对英语专业词汇的影响尤为突出，如 botany（植物学）、phlebotomy（静脉切开放血术）、mathematics（数学）、electron（电子）、aerodynamics（空气动力学）等。其次，拉丁语是古代欧洲科学文化的语言，也有大量拉丁语新词进入英语词汇，如 acupuncture（针灸）、ambulance（救护车）、datum（资料）等。

除此之外，英语专业词汇还不断从其他语言借用来词语丰富自己。例如，来自德语的 autobahn（高速公路），来自西班牙语的 silo（导弹发射井），来自法语的 chiffon（雪纺绸），来自俄语的 sputnik（人造卫星），来自日语的 kamikaze（遥控飞行器），来自意大利语的 stromenti（乐器）等。

7．截断法

截断法，顾名思义，就是截去某单词的一部分而形成新词。

（1）截去末尾部分（或有一些新变化）

advertisement → ad　广告

bicycle → bike　自行车

mathematics → math　数学

（2）截去开头的部分

aeroplane → plane　飞机

omnibus → bus　公交车

telephone → phone　电话

（3）截去开头和末尾的部分

influenza → flu　流感

detective → tec　侦探

3.2　Listening: VR Anatomy

🎧 Section 1

3D Organon VR Anatomy is the world's first fully-featured virtual reality anatomy atlas. It is an immersive self-discovery experience into the human body.

You can manipulate bones, muscles, vessels, organs and other anatomical structures in 3D space. You can examine structures from all angles, read or hear anatomical terminology and study descriptive texts. You can also delve into the body systems, peek under the skin, and see what you are made of.

The new updated version of the app includes the human motion module, with animations of joints and bones. 3D Organon unfolds life-like high resolution 3D models covering every aspect of the human body. The extensive knowledge-base of anatomical definitions and terminology is based on the official Terminologia Anatomica.

The application has been featured in the keynote speech of Mark Zuckerberg, co-founder and CEO of Facebook, in OC3 conference. It has been recommended by leading publications reporting on the future of science, education, and medicine, such as Huffington Post, Scimex, SBS, Futurism, and others.

🎧 Section 2

Educational advantages are the gamification of learning and that students are finding the experience stimulating, engaging and fun. Also, it keeps distractors away due to a high degree of immersion and brings boredom factor out of the classroom.

The 3D models on 3D Organon VR Anatomy can add important cognitive input for understanding key anatomical concepts, leading to an increased retention of knowledge.

Who is 3D Organon Anatomy for?

The app is designed to suit a range of users, from medical and allied-health students to educators, healthcare professionals, patients, artists, and curious minds. It is helping students grasp the challenging subject of anatomy, but also is easily understood by individuals without a medical background. It is an advanced learning tool that could complement any anatomy curriculum and help everyone visualize and explore anatomy.

The application delivers accurate visual and textual information, immediate response time and intuitive navigation. It satisfies the highest standards of medical and scientific accuracy. All anatomical definitions and clinical correlations are written by professors of anatomy and medical professionals.

🎧 Section 3

By using this application you can:

- Explore 15 human body systems with more than 4,000 realistic anatomical structures and organs;
- Grab and move structures in 3D space with life-like precision;
- Easily understand spatial relationships between anatomical structures;
- Zoom in and take a close look at any organ, nerve, vessel, etc.;
- Read and listen anatomical terminology and study descriptive texts;
- Unique stereoscopic presentation of 3D anatomy;
- Inner image of male and female human body designed with precision and aesthetics;
- X-ray mode feature when fading single or multiple structures.

You can get to know the following systems of male and female body:

- Skeletal;
- Connective;
- Muscular;
- Arterial;
- Venous;
- Nervous;
- Lymphatic;
- Heart;
- Respiratory;
- Digestive;
- Endocrine;
- Urinary;
- Reproductive;
- Sensory organs;
- Integumentary (skin).

◆ *Source: https://www.viveport.com/apps/10fc4de2-db6f-49ed-996f-9048e67c509b.*

Listening Exercises

Listen to each section twice, and as you are listening, (a) number the words or expressions in the list on the work sheet by order of their first appearance in the passage you are listening to; (b) check if your numbering is correct—if incorrect, listen to the section again; (c) orally answer the questions about the content of each section.

Unit 3, Section 1

fully-featured	keynote speech	reporting
high resolution	peek	terminology
immersive	recommended	vessels

1. What can the user do with the 3D Organon VR Anatomy atlas? Name three possibilities.

2. What are the anatomical definitions used in the 3D Organon VR Anatomy based on?

3. According to the present description, who recommends this software program?

Unit 3, Section 2

challenging	correlations	intuitive
cognitive	distractors	range
complement	gamification	textual

1. What will help users concentrate on their learning task of exploring the human body?

2. Is the 3D Organon software only intended for specialists?

3. Is this software all that is needed to teach an anatomy curriculum?

Unit 3, Section 3

aesthetics	grab	realistic
arterial	integumentary	skeletal
endocrine	lymphatic	stereoscopic

1. How many human body systems can be explored using this software, and how many anatomical structures?

2. Can you learn the pronunciation of anatomical terms by using this software?

3. Name five of the human body systems presented by this software.

3.3   Writing: Paragraph

在快节奏的阅读时代，如果论文的信息表达不够清晰，就很难吸引读者。论文不能吸引读者主要有以下几方面原因：

- 结构不好；
- 断句不好；
- 大量的长句和长段落；

■ 信息模棱两可或者冗余。

如果读者需要花大量的时间和精力来研读一篇论文，那么他们很可能会放弃阅读。本节关于段落的内容涉及如何将句子有逻辑性地连接起来组成段落，如何将长句变为更易理解的短句。阅读论文时，读者并非一定从头看到尾，可能从任何一个部分（引言、讨论、结论等）开始。每段的第一句话应告诉读者这一段是讲什么的，这样读者可随意跳过此段。每段的最后一句话应该是此段的结论或者告诉读者下一段将讲什么，段落中的句子应该自始至终通过逻辑关系连接，实现由旧信息到新信息的流动。

要记住，在写作时永远将读者放在第一位，站在读者的角度去写。

段落的构成

确定好段落的结构是写好论文关键的一步。段落有长有短，短的可能只有一个句子，长的可能有十多个句子。不论长短，段落的主题必须表达清楚，并且一个段落最好只包含一个主题。

一般而言，一个段落应该包括以下三个主要部分。

（1）主题句（topic sentence），用来阐述段落的核心观点。一般情况下，主题句为段落的第一句，直接点明主题。

（2）论证句（supporting sentence），又称支持句，用来对主题句做具体阐述，主要通过列举事实、范例、原因等阐明主题。

（3）结论句（concluding sentence），用来总结要点，提出供读者思考的一些见解。同时，结论句表明段落的结束，有时也用于引出下一个段落。

段落的写作要点

一般来说，在写每一个段落时必须注意以下两个要点。

（1）一致性。一个段落应阐明一个概念，说明一个问题或一个问题的某一个方面。一个段落都应只讲一个观点。在一段里表述多个观点很难使读者知道此段想表达什么、该记住什么。

（2）连贯性。段落应条理清晰，句子与句子之间的衔接应自然连贯。段落中所描述的主题顺序要合乎逻辑，语言要自然流畅，避免杂乱无章。

段落中的长句改为短句

每当写完一个句子，在大声朗读它的时候如果需要换气，就需要将这个句子改为短句。

一般而言，一个句子不要超过 35 个单词。在书写句子时，尽量多使用句号，少使用逗号，不使用分号和括号。长句如果表达得清晰、易于理解，也可出现在文中。但是如果出现以下情况，请将其改为短句。

■ which + which，一个句子中有两个 which 从句。

■ and + and + and，一个句子中出现了三个及以上 and。

■ , + , + , + , + ,，一个句子中出现五个逗号。

■ also + in addition/furthermore，一个句子中同时出现 also 和 in addition/furthermore。

例句

S1. Using four different methodologies previously used in the literature in separate contexts, each of which gave contradictory results in this study, the meaning of life as seen through the perspective of a typical inhabitant of western Europe was investigated confirming previous research indicating that as a general rule we understand absolutely nothing. (63 words)

S2. Using four different methodologies each of which gave contradictory results, we investigated the meaning of life confirming previous research indicating that we understand absolutely nothing. (25 words)

与 S1 相比，S2 较为简短且更易于理解。

时态与语态

汉语和英语在时态和语态的表示上有很大差异，因此时态与语态也是英文科技论文写作中应重点掌握的内容。

1. 时态

英文科技论文中陈述句所占比例几乎为 100%，这是因为科技英语的显著特点是叙述逻辑上的连贯及表达上的明晰与畅达。作者会避免表露个人感情，避免主观随意性。

英文科技论文中常用的时态有一般现在时、一般过去时、一般将来时和现在完成时。按照惯例，有些时态的表达形式可以与作者所要传达的信息内容形成对应关系。

- 一般现在时：一般现在时在英文科技论文中表述科学定义、定理，对公式的解说以及对图表的说明也多用一般现在时。使用一般现在时的目的在于给人以精确无误的"无时间性"之感，以排除任何可能与时间有牵连的误解，使行文更生动。一般现在时用于已确立的理论、普遍真理，以及具有可重复的实践或操作方法、理论和技术等。在论文中描述研究的目的、研究内容、结果和结论时可用一般现在时。

例句

Action is equal to reaction but it acts in a contrary direction. For every action there is an equal and opposite reaction.

作用力和反作用力大小相等，方向相反。

In practice, time is a relatively easy variable to control.

在实践中，时间是一个相对容易的可控变量。

- 一般过去时：用于描述论文撰写前作者已完成的工作，也可用于表示转述已发表的文献的讨论和研究内容。
- 现在完成时：用于表示某项研究工作已经完成，强调其影响与作用；也可表示该研究或工作到撰写论文时还在持续。
- 一般将来时：主要用于研究设想。

具体到论文的各个部分，大致规则如下。

➢ 摘要：主要为一般过去时，介绍性的陈述可以使用一般现在时。

➢ 引言：主要为一般现在时。

> 方法：一般过去时。
> 结果：一般过去时。
> 讨论：一般现在时。

2．语态

被动语态是 19 世纪以来直到第二次世界大战前英文科技论文中普遍使用的语态。英文科技论文陈述的是客观规律与一般事实，所以一般情况下不使用人称代词作主语，而使用 it 作主语的频率较高。英文科技论文写作中很少用到第一人称。如 I think…，I feel…，I believe…这些说法是主观性的表现，与科技论文书写的客观精神不相符。

过去强调科技论文使用第三人称是认为这样显得客观。而现在的趋势是主张论文要清晰、自然，不必拘泥于主动、被动语态，不强调多用被动语态。因此，现在的科技论文中谓语动词用主动语态的情况越来越多，语句的表达也更为清晰、简洁、有力。

那么，在科技论文写作中，需要表达"我"这一概念时就可以采用灵活多变的方式。如用被动语态，或者用 the author 代表 I，用 the authors 代表 we。此外，还可以用 this study、this report、this paper、this article 等代替第一人称代词。

例句

This paper reports an investigation of this hypothesis.

3.4　Speaking: Conference Presentation—Practice

在开始练习会议报告时，很多人会发现自己的报告时间过长。一般在一开始时报告人都会准备过多的内容。因此，当初步准备好会议报告的内容之后，报告人应再次检查所有内容，并标明必要时可以省略的部分。

做好会议报告最重要的原则之一是说话的速度要慢。对以英语为母语的人而言，适当的速度为每分钟不超过一百个英文单词。对母语非英语的人而言，适当的速度可能还要更慢。因此，如果准备做十五分钟的报告，那么报告的内容就不要超过一千五百个英文单词。

在正式报告之前，要反复练习。多练习可以使我们对自己的演讲能力更有自信，也可以使我们在做会议报告时以更有效、更具说服力的方式来表达报告的内容。

练习做会议报告的方法有很多。较简单的方法是在家里照着镜子练习，最好可以录音，在练习完毕时可以试听自己的报告内容，并找出需要改进的地方。还可以借助录像，录下自己在练习会议报告时的情形，然后再观看录像。不论是听录音或看录像，报告人都应该注意是否有些地方暂停太久，讲解不同部分时过渡是否自然。另外，报告人应该特别注意自己是否常常发出一些如"哦""啊"等无意义的声音，或常常重复如 OK、good 等虚词。如果是，则应尽量去除这些口头语。最后，注意自己是否常常有些重复的手势，或表现出其他可能扰乱听众注意力的坏习惯。

此外，在练习会议报告时，报告人应该特别注意下列两点。

■ 多练习报告的不同部分或小标题之间的衔接与过渡。不同小标题间的衔接应清楚、自然、通顺、合理。在做转接时，报告人可以多利用如 now let me describe…，以及 next, let's look at…等句型，让听众紧紧跟随报告的进展。然而，这些句型并不是必需的。例如，在介绍实验结果时，直接说 here are the results of the first test，也无可厚非。

■ 可以想出几种不同的表达方式重述报告的重点。在会议报告中，报告人需要多次重复自己的主要论点，例如，在引言中叙述一次，在提供证据以支持论点之前或之后叙述一次，在最后进行总结时再叙述一次。如果在每次重述同一个论点时都使用同样的句子，听众就会觉得报告的内容单调、枯燥。因此，对于报告的主要论点，报告人应多准备几种不同的表达方式。

Unit 4   Biomaterials

4.1   Text: Biomaterials

Nature has always been a source of inspiration for technical developments, but only in recent years have materials scientists started to consider the complex hierarchical structure of natural materials as a model for the development of new types of high-performance engineering materials.[1] It is by no means obvious how the lessons learned from biological materials can be applied to the design of new engineering materials.[2] The reasons for this difficulty are some striking differences in the design strategies that are common in engineering and the ways in which natural materials are constructed. First, the choice of elements is by far greater for the engineer. Elements such as iron, chromium and nickel are only trace elements in biological tissues and are not used in metallic form, in contrast to their use in different types of steel, for example.[3] A second difference is in the way that materials are actually made. Whereas the engineer takes a "top-down" approach, selecting a material to fabricate a part according to an established goal and an exact design plan, natural structures develop in the opposite way (that is, "bottom up").[4] Both the material and the whole organism (a plant or an animal) grow according to the principles of biologically controlled self-assembly. This provides control over the structure of the material at all times and levels of hierarchy, and it is the key to the outstanding success with which composites are used as structural materials in nature. Therefore, many crucial features of biological materials are worth understanding. These include their hierarchical structure, their remarkable fracture resistance, their multifunctional or adaptive properties, and their self-healing capacity.

To derive useful biologically inspired strategies in materials science, it is not sufficient simply to observe naturally occurring structures. Organisms have to cope with a multitude of environmental constraints that typically differ greatly from the boundary conditions to be met by materials developed for technological application.[5] In an animal or a plant, a material evolved to serve a mechanical function also needs to fulfill many other criteria. For example, it may have to grow under temperature, pressure and pH conditions indispensable for the existence of life. Also, the material's constituents have to be available in the habitat of the species in question. Furthermore, the material may have to serve not only structural functions but also functions needed for camouflage, signalling, defence against bacteria and parasites, and so on. The constraints on the manufacture of an engineering material are drastically different. They include consumer acceptance, compatibility with other technical systems, and the time and cost of manufacturing. Whereas the engineer generally knows the constraints and selects a material appropriately, biomimetic materials science requires the study of a pre-existing natural material that represents the solution to an unknown, multifaceted problem, which makes the transfer of principles to materials engineering more difficult. The relationship between the function of the biological material and its structure and composition has to be fully established before any principle useful in materials science can be extracted.[6] As a result, there is no biomimetic materials research without proper biological research, including a thorough analysis of what a material is made for under the conditions of the organism's species-specific behaviour and ecological situation. A consequence of this is that although the study of materials in organisms may inspire radically new materials designs, it does not lead to rapid solutions in materials engineering.

The combination of materials science and biology also contributes significantly to the biological understanding of organisms by helping to establish structure-function relationships: developing mathematical or technical models of biological systems helps to clarify the function of their components. It may even allow quantitative predictions about the evolutionary role and relative importance of certain parameters in the development of particular functions enforced by natural selection.

Glossary

chromium [ˈkrəʊmiəm]	*n.* 铬
metallic [mɪˈtælɪk]	*adj.* 金属的
fabricate [ˈfæbrɪkeɪt]	*vt.* 制造
composite [ˈkɒmpəzɪt]	*n.* 复合材料
constraint [kənˈstreɪnt]	*n.* 限制
indispensable [ˌɪndɪˈspensəbəl]	*adj.* 不可缺少的
constituent [kənˈstɪtʃuənt]	*n.* 成分
habitat [ˈhæbɪtæt]	*n.* 生境、栖生地
camouflage [ˈkæməˈflɑːʒ]	*n.* 伪装
drastically [ˈdræstɪkli]	*adv.* 彻底地
biomimetic [ˌbaɪəʊmɪˈmetɪk]	*adj.* 仿生的

Technical Terms

hierarchical structure	层次结构
trace element	微量元素
fracture resistance	抗断裂性
in question	讨论中的
species-specific behavior	物种特异行为

Notes

1. Nature has always been a source of inspiration for technical developments, but only in recent years have materials scientists started to consider the complex hierarchical structure of natural materials as a model for the development of new types of high-performance engineering materials.

自然界一直是技术发展的灵感源泉，但直到近年来，材料科学家才开始以天然材料的复杂层次结构为模型，开发新型高性能工程材料。

分析：…in recent years have materials scientists…中 have 提至主语前，属于倒装句中的部分倒装。部分倒装是指将该句中谓语的一部分，如助动词或情态动词，倒装于主语之前。

2. It is by no means obvious how the lessons learned from biological materials can be applied to the design of new engineering materials.

还不明确的是，如何将从生物材料中汲取的知识应用于设计新型工程材料。

分析：by no means，意为"并没有，并不"。

句中 it 作形式主语，没有实际意义，指代的是后面的 how the lessons…。

3. Elements such as iron, chromium and nickel are only trace elements in biological tissues and are not used in metallic form, in contrast to their use in different types of steel, for example.

诸如铁、铬和镍等元素只是生物组织中的微量元素，且不以金属形式起作用，这与它们用在不同类型钢材中不同。

分析：in contrast to 意为"与……形成对照"。

4. Whereas the engineer takes a "top-down" approach, selecting a material to fabricate a part according to an established goal and an exact design plan, natural structures develop in the opposite way (that is, "bottom up").

工程师采用"自上而下"的方法，根据既定目标和精确的设计计划来选择材料制造零件，而自然结构则以相反的方式发展（即"自下而上"）。

分析：whereas 意为"然而"，用于比较或对比两个事实。

5. Organisms have to cope with a multitude of environmental constraints that typically differ greatly from the boundary conditions to be met by materials developed for technological application.

生物体必须应对多种环境限制，这些限制通常与为技术应用而开发的材料所要满足的边界条件有很大不同。

分析：to be met by…不定式作定语，与其被修饰的词在逻辑上为被动关系。

6. The relationship between the function of the biological material and its structure and composition has to be fully established before any principle useful in materials science can be extracted.

在推导出任何可用于材料科学的原理之前，必须完全确立生物材料的功能与其结构和组成之间的关系。

分析：useful in materials…形容词短语作后置定语，修饰 principle。

Translation Skills：外来科技术语的翻译方法

由于科技英语自身专业性强、知识更新速度快，在科技英语的翻译过程中，常常会涉及许多外来科技术语的翻译。科技术语是准确地表示科技领域的某一概念的词语，用来记录和表达各种现象、过程、特性、关系、状态。它集中反映了科学概念和科技内容，是科技信息的主要载体，也是科学论述的必要条件。翻译外来科技术语主要有意译、音译、半音半意、形译、直译等方法。

1. 意译法

意译法是指按照原词所表达的具体事物和概念译出科学概念，基本上采用照搬源语内容和意义的方法，来创建目标语中没有的新术语，以表达新的概念。这样创造出的新术语便于读者接受和理解。例如，

videophone	可视电话
holography	全息投影
E-mail	电子邮件
clock frequency	时钟频率
gravity	地球引力
air conditioner	空调
dial balance	刻度天平
data base	数据库
think tank	智囊团
garbage	无用信息

2. 音译法

音译法就是根据英语单词的发音译成读音与原词大致相同的汉字。音译法一方面主要用来翻译以人名命名的科学度量单位，而这类常用的科学度量单位大多可以进一步简化，只音译一个音节。例如，

Volt	伏特（电压单位，简称伏）
Bit	比特（度量信息的单位，二进制位）
Lux	勒克斯（照明单位，简称勒）
Joule	焦耳（功或能的单位，简称焦）
Ohm	欧姆（电阻单位，简称欧）

另一方面，音译法可以用来翻译某些新发明的材料或产品的名称（尤其在起初时），如材料、产品、军事装备、药品等。例如，

nylon	尼龙
morphine	吗啡
Vaseline	凡士林
sofa	沙发
Benz	奔驰
radar	雷达
Aspirin	阿司匹林

一般来说，音译比意译容易，但不如意译更能够明确地表达术语的含义。因此，有些音译词经过一段时间后往往会被意译词所取代，或者同时使用。例如，

laser	镭射→激光
vitamin	维他命→维生素
penicillin	盘尼西林→青霉素

3. 半音半意法

在科技术语的翻译中，有些术语采用一部分音译，另一部分意译的方法。

有些词以音译为主，在词首或词尾加上表意的词。例如，

moto-cycle	摩托车
valve body	阀体
topology	拓扑学
logic circuit	逻辑电路

有些词是把一部分音译，另一部分意译。例如，

Morse code	莫尔斯码
radariste	雷达专家
neon lamp	霓虹灯
Taylor formula	泰勒公式
Norton gear	诺顿齿轮

4. 形译法

科技英语中，常常利用字母的形象来为形状相似的物体定名，对于这类字母，可采用形译法。常见的形译法有三种。

（1）从汉语中选取能够表达原字母形象的字词来翻译。例如，

I-bar	工字钢
U-bend	马蹄弯头
V-slot	三角形槽

（2）保留原字母不译，在该字母后加"形"字。例如，

A-frame	A 形架
M-wing	M 形机翼
A-bedlate	A 形底座
C-clamp	C 形夹
O-ring	O 形环

（3）保留原字母不译，以字母代表一种概念。例如，

P-region	P 区（电子不足区）
L-electron	L 层电子（原子核外第二层电子）
X-ray	X 射线

5. 直译法

由于各国交流日益频繁，有的新词还未来得及找到合适的翻译，便已经原样流传开来。商标、牌号、型号和表示特定意义的字母均可不译，直接使用原文，只译普通名词。例如，

B-52 E bomber	B-52 E 轰炸机
Kubota Mobile Crane Model KM-150	库宝塔 KM-150 型移动式起重机
PC	PC（个人计算机）
YaHoo	YaHoo（美国著名的互联网门户网站）
XO	XO（一种法国产白兰地酒）

4.2   Listening: Biomaterials

Section 1

A biomaterial is any substance that has been engineered to interact with biological systems for a medical purpose—either a therapeutic (treat, augment, repair or replace a tissue function of the body) or a diagnostic one. As a science, biomaterials is about fifty years old. The study of biomaterials is called biomaterials science or biomaterials engineering. It has experienced steady and strong growth over its history, with many companies investing large amounts of money into the development of new products. Biomaterials science encompasses elements of medicine, biology, chemistry, tissue engineering and materials science.

Note that a biomaterial is different from a biological material, such as bone, which is produced by a biological system. Additionally, care should be exercised in defining a biomaterial as biocompatible, since it is application-specific. A biomaterial that is biocompatible or suitable for one application may not be biocompatible for another.

Section 2

Biomaterials can be derived either from nature or synthesized in the laboratory using a variety of chemical approaches utilizing metallic components, polymers, ceramics or composite materials. They are often used and/or adapted for a medical application, and thus comprises whole or part of a living structure or biomedical device which performs, augments, or replaces a natural function. Such functions may be relatively passive, like being used for a heart valve, or may be bioactive with a more interactive functionality such as hydroxy-apatite coated hip implants. Biomaterials are also used every day in dental applications, surgery, and drug delivery. For example, a construct with impregnated pharmaceutical products can be placed into the body, which permits the prolonged release of a drug over an extended period of time. A biomaterial may also be an autograft, allograft or xenograft used as a transplant material.

Biomaterials are used in:
- joint replacements;
- bone plates;
- intraocular lenses (IOLs) for eye surgery;
- bone cement;
- artificial ligaments and tendons;
- dental implants for tooth fixation;
- blood vessel prostheses;
- heart valves;
- skin repair devices (artificial tissue);
- cochlear replacements;

- contact lenses;
- breast implants;
- drug delivery mechanisms;
- sustainable materials;
- vascular grafts;
- stents;
- nerve conduits;
- surgical sutures, clips, and staples for wound closure;
- pins and screws for fracture stabilisation;
- surgical mesh.

🎧 Section 3

Biomaterials must be compatible with the body, and there are often issues of biocompatibility which must be resolved before a product can be placed on the market and used in a clinical setting. Because of this, biomaterials are usually subjected to the same requirements as those undergone by new drug therapies.

All manufacturing companies are also required to ensure traceability of all of their products so that if a defective product is discovered, others in the same batch may be traced.

Compatibility.

Biocompatibility is related to the behavior of biomaterials in various environments under various chemical and physical conditions. The term may refer to specific properties of a material without specifying where or how the material is to be used. For example, a material may elicit little or no immune response in a given organism, and may or may not be able to integrate with a particular cell type or tissue. The ambiguity of this term reflects the ongoing development of insights into how biomaterials interact with the human body and eventually how those interactions determine the clinical success of a medical device (such as pacemaker or hip replacement). Modern medical devices and prostheses are often made of more than one material—so it might not always be sufficient to talk about the biocompatibility of a specific material.

◆ *Source: https://en.wikipedia.org/wiki/Biomaterial.*

Listening Exercises

Listen to each section twice, and as you are listening, (a) number the words or expressions in the list on the work sheet by order of their first appearance in the passage you are listening to; (b) check if your numbering is correct—if incorrect, listen to the section again; (c) orally answer the questions about the content of each section.

Unit 4, Section 1

biocompatible	diagnostic	investing
biological	encompasses	suitable
chemistry	interact	therapeutic

1. What are the two main purposes of biomaterials?

2. What sciences contribute to the study of biomaterials?

3. Is any biomaterial always suitable for all applications?

Unit 4, Section 2

autograft	intraocular	passive
cochlear replacements	mesh	polymers
impregnated	nerve conduits	prostheses

1. What materials are use to synthesize biomaterials?

2. Give an example of a passive medical device and an example of a bioactive medical device.

3. Name five uses of biomaterials.

Unit 4, Section 3

ambiguity	eventually	specific
behavior	insights	traceability
elicit	issues	undergone by

1. How is the quality of biomaterials assured?

2. Can the biocompatibility of biomaterials be determined immediately?

3. Why is it not sufficient to talk about the biocompatibility of one specific material?

4.3　Writing: Article

撰写英文科技论文的第一步是推敲结构。一种简单有效的方法是采用 IMRaD
（Introduction，Materials and Methods，Results，and Discussion）形式，这是英文科技论文通
用的结构。IMRaD 结构的逻辑体现在它能依次回答以下问题。

- ■ Introduction（引言）：研究问题是什么？
- ■ Materials and Methods（材料和方法）：怎样研究这个问题？
- ■ Results（结果）：发现了什么？
- ■ Discussion（讨论）：这些发现意味着什么？

在按照这个结构整体规划论文时，有一个方法值得借鉴，即剑桥大学爱席比教授提出
的"概念图"。首先在一张大纸上（A3 或 A4 纸，横放）写下论文题目（事先定好题目很重
要），然后根据 IMRaD 的结构确定基本的段落主题，把它们写在不同的方框内。科研人员可
以记录任何闪现在脑海中的可以包括在该部分的内容，诸如段落标题、图表、需要进一步阐
述的观点等，把它们写在方框附近的圈内，并用箭头标示它们所属的方框。画概念图的阶段
也是自由思考的阶段，在此过程中不必拘泥于细节。哪些东西需要写进论文，还需要做哪些
工作（是找到某文献的原文，还是补画一张图表，或者需要再查找某个参考文献）等问题都
可体现在概念图中。当需要再加进一个段落时，就在概念图中添加一个新方框。如果发现原
来的顺序需做调整，那么就用箭头标示新的顺序。绘制概念图的过程看似儿童游戏，但意义
重大。它可以提供自由思考的空间，并通过图示的方式记录思维发展的过程。这便是写论文

的第一步：从整体考虑论文结构，思考各种组织论文的方法，准备好所需的资料，并随时记录出现的新想法。采用这个方法，不论正式下笔时从哪一部分写起，都能够做到大局不乱。

英文科技论文的基本格式

一篇完整的英文科技论文通常包括以下部分：

- Title（论文题目）；
- Author(s)（作者姓名）；
- Affiliation(s) and address(es)（联系方式）；
- Abstract（摘要）；
- Keywords（关键词）；
- Body（正文）；
- Acknowledgements（致谢，可空缺）；
- References（参考文献）；
- Appendix（附录，可空缺）；
- Resume（作者简介，视刊物而定）。

其中正文为论文的主体部分，分为若干章节。一篇完整的科技论文的正文部分由以下内容构成：

- Introduction（引言/概述）；
- Materials and Methods（材料和方法）；
- Results（结果）；
- Discussion（讨论）；
- Conclusion（结论/总结）。

写作顺序

科技论文的撰写不一定要按照上述顺序书写，一是很多人觉得引言很难写，二是事实上先写其他的章节也无妨。例如，可以先写材料和方法章节（材料和方法章节通常比其他章节容易下手），然后再写结果章节。结果章节写完后，作者会对整个论文的内容或重点有更深入的了解，这时再写引言或许会容易一些。研究报告的讨论及结论章节是特别重要的两部分，在这两章中作者不仅要对自己的研究结果提出完整的解释，而且要说明这些结果有什么意义和内涵。有一位专业编辑曾表示：即使论文所提出的研究结果很有意思，但是只要讨论章节写得不够完整或稍有瑕疵，也很可能会被退稿。所以在写作过程中，一定要重视讨论章节和结论章节，要让自己有足够的时间慢慢琢磨和修改这两部分的内容。

在准备把研究论文投稿到专业期刊时，一定要首先查阅该期刊编辑对于论文的组织及格式的说明，而且应翻阅几篇该期刊曾出版的论文，以便了解其规定的格式，如摘要格式、参考文献格式、图表格式，以及关于论文篇幅及图表数量的限制等。

4.4　Speaking: Conference Presentation—Presentation

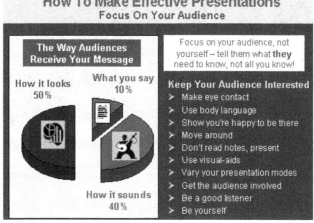

（资料来源：https://ventures.powweb.com/business_guide/crosscuttings/presentations_main.html）

图 4.1　如何做有效的报告

从图 4.1 中可以看到，听众对于报告的兴趣，90%取决于报告人如何组织表述、如何演讲。报告内容要逻辑清晰、重点突出，在做报告时体态要自然大方。

1．语言

语言要清楚，语调要自然。在做报告时吐字要清晰，尽量用简单的字词与表达方式，而且语速应缓慢而有节奏感。切勿认为一定要用很复杂的语言才能获得听众的认可。如果会议报告内容清楚，组织有条理，而且研究内容本身有一定的专业水平，那么听众自然就会认可，不会去注意英语句子是否略微简单。

在报告中应避免生硬的、不自然的句子结构。在论文中看起来稍显生硬的句子，在报告中会听起来更不自然。例如，在介绍某个图表中的数据时，应避免如 it is shown in this figure that…或 it can be seen from this figure that…等被动语句，而应简单地说 this figure shows that...或 from this figure, we can see that…。

另外，最好能够训练语速的节奏感，根据内容适当变化语速和音量。紧张或没有经验的报告人更容易在做报告时语速加快。试着放慢语速，并且通过增加一些停顿来达到强调的效果。

2．身体语言亲切自然

- 面部表情放松而和谐，与听众有眼神的交流。在环视全场时，可以寻找亲切的面孔来缓解紧张情绪。每次只与一位听众进行目光交流，而且目光在每个人身上停留持续 5 秒或者持续到一个意图表达完整之后再离开。做报告的重点是把要表达的内容传递给听众，与听众有目光的交流可以使报告人更可信、更真诚。
- 身体姿态自信、自然。姿势端正有利于呼吸和发音顺畅。无须事先计划手势，手势应该是所要传达的信息的延伸，事先计划的手势看起来会很不自然，刻意为之还会和其他自然的肢体语言不搭配。建议多用手掌少用手指，利用手势表达情感也不必太多，否则会显得紧张。如果非常紧张，可以握拳，手自然下垂即可。

● 可以在开放的空间走动，有效地贴近听众，但是不要背对听众。

● 着装最好是正装，演讲时穿着得体、正式的衣服，也会更自信。

3. 有趣、富有激情的报告

要让听众感受到报告人的激情和对所讲内容的热爱与确定。将激情注入报告中，乐在其中。不要读幻灯片上的内容，回头看幻灯片会打断报告人的思路，也间接地告诉听众报告人根本就不理解自己要讲的内容，从而对报告失去信心和兴趣。在用英文做报告时，应尽量细心准备，并多练习英文演讲技巧。报告中不要担心自己的语言能力不够好。只要认真准备，内容清楚、有趣、充实，即使在英文表述方面有些小问题，仍然可以获得听众的肯定。

此外，在做报告的前一天晚上应保证充足的睡眠。如果身体出现疲惫感，则可能影响报告的效果。

4. 将会议报告看作提高自己和同行交流的机会

报告人应享受做报告的过程，将会议报告看作提高自己和同行交流的机会。如果已经精心准备了，在做报告时只需专心按照自己的计划来进行报告即可。把自己的研究成果与同行交流是一件很愉快的事情。

5. 将听众视为自己的朋友

在做报告时，应该提醒自己：听众并不是评委，他们不是在时刻判断我们的对错。听众是和我们一样的人，他们来听报告是为了进行学术交流和培养人际关系。如果可能的话，可在做报告前找机会与部分参会者见面、聊天。这样我们就更能让自己放松，把做报告看成和听众谈话一样（而事实上，做报告本来就如同和听众谈话一样）。

6. 常常做小结

在报告的每一部分结束时，应对该部分的重点做总结。此外，如果报告很长，可以让听众有机会提问题。但是，听众发问的时间不能过长，以免影响整个报告的进行。若对某个问题需要做很长、很详细的解答，则应表示暂时保留此问题，在报告完毕后再讨论。

Unit 5　Tissue Engineering

5.1　Text: Tissue Engineering

Tissue engineering can be defined as the application of scientific principles to the design, construction, modification, growth, and maintenance of living tissues.[1] Tissue engineering can be divided into two broad categories: (1) *in vitro* construction of bioartificial tissues from cells isolated by enzymatic dissociation of donor tissue, and (2) *in vivo* alteration of cell growth and function. The first category of applications includes bioartificial tissues (i.e., tissues which are composed of natural and synthetic substances) to be used as an alternative to organ transplantation. Besides their potential clinical use, reconstructed organs may also be used as tools to study complex tissue functions and morphogenesis *in vitro*. For tissue engineering *in vivo*, the objective is to alter the growth and function of cells *in situ*, an example being the use of implanted polymeric tubes to promote the growth and reconnection of damaged nerves. Some representative examples of applications of tissue engineering currently being pursued are listed in Table 5.1.

Table 5.1　Representative Applications of Tissue Engineering

Application	Examples
Implantable device	Endothelialized vascular grafts
Extracorporeal device	Bone and cartilage implants
Cell production	Bioartificial skin
In situ tissue growth and repair	Bioartificial pancreatic islets
	Neurotransmitter-secreting cells
	Bioartificial liver
	Hematopoiesis *in vitro*
	Nerve regeneration
	Artificial skin

Conceptually, bioartificial tissues involve three-dimensional structures with cell masses that are orders of magnitude greater than that used in traditional two-dimensional cell culture techniques.[2] In addition, bioartificial organ technology often involves highly differentiated somatic and parenchymal cells isolated from normal tissues. In the bioartificial structures, the tissue compartments must be scaled to mimic nutrient transport existent within natural capillary beds found in the body.[3] Generally, these *in vivo* beds are composed of 100 mm thick tissue slabs sandwiched by vasculature. Thus, the microenvironment of *ex vivo* bioartificial devices must also maintain these limitations in order to provide appropriate concentrations of nutrients to tissue cultures. Once this *ex vivo* capillary scaling is achieved，then more advanced engineered devices must be designed in order to support larger cell masses. One such design is a bioreactor that maintains appropriate radial scaling parameters while longitudinally extending the cellular space.[4] Additionally, for automated cell cultures and manufactured devices, the scaling up (or down for individual cell analysis) must maintain correct proportions of nutrient and biomass interactions; therefore, based upon need, distinctive scaling parameters are necessary for unique applications. Some of these applications are discussed with a few examples below: (1) The reconstitution of physical (mass transfer) and biological (soluble and insoluble signals) microenvironments for the development of tissue function; (2) To overcome scale-up problems in order to generate cellular microenvironments that are clinically meaningful; (3) The system automation to perform on clinically meaningful scales; (4) The implementation of devices in clinical settings, with cell handling and preservation procedures that are required for cell therapies.

Glossary

modification [ˌmɒdɪfɪˈkeɪʃən]	*n.* 修改，修正；改变
maintenance [ˈmeɪntənəns]	*n.* 保持
alternative [ɔːlˈtɜːnətɪv]	*n.* 二中择一
morphogenesis [ˌmɔːfəˈdʒɛnəsɪs]	*n.* 形态发生，形态形成
extracorporeal [ˌekstrəkɔːˈpɔːrɪəl]	*adj.* 身体外的
cartilage [ˈkɑːtɪlɪdʒ]	*n.* 软骨，软骨结构
hematopoiesis [ˌhimətopɔɪˈisɪs]	*n.* 造血作用，生血作用
conceptually [kənˈseptʃuəli]	*adv.* 概念地
differentiated [ˌdɪfəˈrenʃieɪtɪd]	*adj.* 分化的
mimic [ˈmɪmɪk]	*vt.* 模仿，仿真
sandwich [ˈsænwɪdʒ]	*vt.* 夹入，夹在中间
vasculature [ˈvæskjələˌtʃə]	*n.* 脉管系统
microenvironment [ˌmaikroɪnˈvaɪrənmənt]	*n.* 微环境
concentration [ˌkɒnsənˈtreɪʃən]	*n.* 浓度
bioreactor [ˌbaioriˈæktə]	*n.* 生物反应器
longitudinally [lɒndʒɪˈtjuːdɪnəli]	*adv.* 长度上，纵向地

Technical Terms

tissue engineering	组织工程
in vitro	离体的
bioartificial tissues	人工生物组织
enzymatic dissociation	酶解离
donor tissue	供体组织
in vivo	体内的
synthetic substances	合成物质

organ transplantation	器官移植
reconstructed organs	重建器官
complex tissue	复合组织
in situ	在原位置，在原处
implanted polymeric tube	植入聚合物管
endothelialized vascular grafts	内皮血管移植
bioartificial pancreatic islets	人工胰岛
neurotransmitter-secreting cell	神经递质分泌细胞
nerve regeneration	神经再生
somatic and parenchymal cell	体细胞和实质细胞
nutrient transport	营养物运输，养分运输
ex vivo	体外的
capillary scaling	毛细管缩放
cell masses	细胞团
radial scaling parameter	径向缩放参数
biomass interactions	生物相互作用
mass transfer	传质

Notes

1. Tissue engineering can be defined as the application of scientific principles to the design，construction, modification, growth, and maintenance of living tissues.

组织工程学可以定义为应用科学原理设计、构造、修复、培养和维持生命组织的学科。

分析：something can be defined as…为被动语态，主动语态为…define something as…。

2. Conceptually, bioartificial tissues involve three-dimensional structures with cell masses that are orders of magnitude greater than that used in traditional two-dimensional cell culture techniques.

从概念上讲，生物人造组织涉及的三维结构在细胞团的数量级上要比传统的二维细胞培养技术大得多。

分析：sth. are orders of magnitude greater than sth. 是一种比较结构，其结构为比较级形容词＋than＋比较成分，表示"比……更……"。

3. In the bioartificial structures, the tissue compartments must be scaled to mimic nutrient transport existent within natural capillary beds found in the body.

在生物人造结构中，组织区室必须被缩放以模拟身体中自然毛细管床中的营养物运输。

分析：found in the body 是后置定语作修饰成分，修饰 nutrient transport。

4. One such design is a bioreactor that maintains appropriate radial scaling parameters while longitudinally extending the cellular space.

生物反应器就采用这样一种设计，它能在保持适当的径向伸缩参数的同时纵向扩展细胞空间。

分析：that 引导限定性定语从句，修饰宾语 bioreactor。

Translation Skills：数词的表示与翻译

1．数词的表示

（1）常用数词的表示

thousands of	成千上万的
hundreds of	数以百计的
decades of	几十年的
ten to one	十比一
nine cases out of ten	十有八九
fifty-fifty	平分
a long hundred	一百多
twos and threes	三三两两
one or two	少许
two over three	三分之二
second to none	第一
last but one	倒数第二
a decade of	十个
a score of	二十个
a dozen of	十二个

（2）分数的表示

常用形式：分子（基数词）/分母（序数词一般为复数，当分子小于或等于 1 时用单数）。例如，

one fifth	五分之一
three fourths/three quarters	四分之三
a/one half	二分之一

🍃例句

Only <u>one fifth</u> of air consists of oxygen.

氧气只占空气的 <u>1/5</u>。

专业英语中经常用到以下两种形式（一般表示较小的分数）。

■ 分子：基数词＋part(s)

  分母：per 或 in a 或 in＋阿拉伯数字

  十亿分之六：6 parts per billion

         6 parts in a billion

         6 parts per 1,000,000,000

■ 分子：a/an＋序数词＋part

  分母：per 或 in a 或 in＋阿拉伯数字

  十亿分之三：a third part in 1,000,000,000

         a third part per billion

a third part in a billion

（3）小数的表示

常用形式：小数用基数词表示，以小数点为界，小数点左边的数字为整数，小数点右边的数字为小数，二者分开读。小数点读作"point"，0 读作"zero"或"o [ou]"，整数部分为零时可以不读，小数点后的数字必须一一读出。

0.5 读作 zero point five 或 point five

26.66 读作 twenty-six point six six

（4）百分数的表示

百分数由 percent 表示，应用时常与 by 连用。

0.65% 读作 zero point six five percent

48% 读作 forty-eight percent

例句

Sales of medical devices have increased by <u>30 percent</u> in recent years。

近几年医疗器械的销售增长了<u>百分之三十</u>。

2．数量增加的翻译

（1）句型：be n times as + 形容词（或副词）+ as…；be n times + 比较级 + than；be + 比较级 + than + 名词 + by n times；be n times + 名词；be + 比较级 + by a factor of n。可译成"是……的 n 倍""n 倍于"或"比……大 (n-1) 倍"。

例句

The oxygen atom is <u>16 times heavier than</u> the hydrogen atom.

氧原子的重量<u>是</u>氢原子<u>的 16 倍</u>。

Because DNA replication precedes the physical division of the cell，there is a period during which the cellular material has <u>twice the normal amount</u> of DNA.

由于 DNA 复制先于细胞的物理分裂，在细胞物质中有一段时期的 DNA 含量<u>是正常数量的 2 倍</u>。

（2）句型：as + 形容词（或副词）+ again as；again as + 形容词（或副词）+ as。可译成"是……的 2 倍"或"比……多（大、长……）1 倍"。如果 again 前加 half，则表示"是……的 1.5 倍"或"比……多（大、长……）半倍"。

例句

This wire <u>is as long again as</u> that one.

这根金属线的长度<u>是</u>那根<u>的 2 倍</u>。

The amount left was estimated to <u>be again as much as</u> all the zinc that has been mined.

当时估计，剩余的锌储量<u>是</u>已开采量<u>的 2 倍</u>。

The resistance of aluminum <u>is</u> approximately <u>half again as great as</u> that of copper for the same dimensions.

尺寸相同时，铝的电阻约<u>为</u>铜<u>的 1.5 倍</u>。

（3）用带有"增大"意思的动词（increase、rise、grow 等）和含有数词的词语配合。句型有：动词 + n times；动词 + by + n times；动词 + to + n times；动词 + n-fold；动词 + by a factor of + n。可译成"增加到 n 倍"或"增加了 (n-1) 倍"。

例句

The strength of the attraction will <u>increase by four times</u> if the distance between the original charges is reduced by half.

如果原电荷的距离缩短一半，则引力就增大到原来的 4 倍。

Circular folds on the inner luminal surface <u>increase</u> the surface area <u>by threefold</u>, villi <u>increase</u> the surface area <u>by tenfold</u>, and microvilli (which constitute the brush border) <u>increase</u> the surface area <u>by twentyfold</u>.

内腔表面的圆形褶皱使表面积增加了 <u>2 倍</u>，绒毛使表面积增加了 <u>9 倍</u>，微绒毛（构成刷状边界）使表面积增加了 <u>19 倍</u>。

Therefore, the total surface area is <u>increased by 600-fold</u> relative to a plain tube.

因此，总表面积增加为普通管的 <u>600 倍</u>。

If X is doubled, Y is <u>increased by a factor of 4</u>.

若 X 增加到 2 倍，则 Y <u>增加到 4 倍</u>。

（4）用表示倍数的动词表示量的增加。例如，double 可译成"增加 1 倍""翻一番"或"是……的 2 倍"；triple 可译成"增加 2 倍"或"增加到 3 倍"；quadruple 可译成"增加 3 倍"或"翻两番"。

例句

As the high voltage was abruptly <u>tripled</u>, all the electrical appliances burnt.

由于高压突然增加了 <u>2 倍</u>，电器都烧坏了。

The new airport will <u>double</u> the capacity of the existing one.

新机场是现有机场容量<u>的 2 倍</u>。

3. 数量减少的翻译

在表达数量减少时，中英文有所不同，翻译时要注意中英文的表达差异。

（1）英文说"减少……倍"，而中文说"减少百分之……"。

例句

The presence of surfactant in the fluid <u>decreases</u> the surface tension <u>by a factor of 10</u>, and also decreases the pressure in the liquid film, allowing the alveoli to remain inflated with less effort from the chest wall.

液体表面的表面活性剂的存在使表面张力<u>降低</u>为原来<u>的 1/10</u>，同时也降低了液体薄膜的压力，使得肺泡在胸腔壁的作用下保持膨胀。

（2）表示"减少一半"时，英文有多种不同的句型和表达方法，翻译时应多加注意。

例句

The new electronic device <u>shortened</u> the circuit <u>by half</u>.

新型电子装置使线路缩短了<u>一半</u>。

This kind of film <u>is twice thinner than</u> ordinary paper, but its quality is good.

这种薄膜的厚度只是普通纸张<u>的一半</u>，可是质量很好。

The laptop <u>is</u> only <u>half as heavy as</u> the old one.

这台笔记本电脑比旧型号的要<u>轻一半</u>。

（3）表示"一般意义上的减少"，英文表达非常灵活。

例句

The half-life of this technetium isotope is short (6 hours), so the radioactivity is <u>cut in half</u> every six hours and therefore does not last long after injection into the body.

这种锝同位素的半衰期很短（6 小时），所以放射性每 6 小时<u>减弱一半</u>，因此注入人体后不会持续太久。

The loss of metal <u>has been reduced to less than 30%</u>.

金属损耗<u>减少到了百分之三十以下</u>。

The ordinary smelting time <u>has been cut by one-fourth</u>.

在通常情况下，提炼时间<u>缩短了四分之一</u>。

5.2　Listening: Tissue Engineering

Section 1

NANTONG, CHINA—Mounted to the entrance of the Jiangsu Key Laboratory of Neuroregeneration is a plaque listing two dozen grants—a total of $2.87 million over 18 years, impressive for a lab in the somewhat obscure Nantong University here, a few hours' drive from Shanghai. A sparkling 4000-square meter complex outfitted with millions of dollars' worth of equipment, as well as a kitchen, a recreation room, lockers and shower facilities, is an even greater testament to the success of the lab's director, Gu Xiaosong. As an expert in peripheral nerve regeneration, he's pushed to make neuroregeneration "a distinguishing characteristic of our school." But in some regards, Gu's lab is not that unusual. It is one of dozens to capitalize on a recent Chinese government push in tissue engineering. "Chinese leaders see tissue engineering as a promising area for innovation," says Cui Fuzhai, a bone and brain tissue engineering specialist at Tsinghua University in Beijing, "They feel that it is important to the economy—that it has clear applications."

Section 2

In recent years, China's national grant programs have singled out this field, along with other aspects of biomaterials research, for growth. From 1999 to 2009, according to a recent analysis by the Boston-based technology consulting firm Lux Research, more than $80 million from various government channels went to tissue engineering and stem cell research in the country. While the government tends not to release funding totals for specific research areas, intensive government investment in stem cells didn't pick up until 2011, says Ma Zhun, an analyst with Lux Research in Shanghai. With calls for the Chinese biomedical materials industry to quintuple its share of the global market by 2050, such funding will almost certainly increase in the decades to come. Chinese tissue engineering research dates back to the 1990s, as the field was coming into its own internationally. Chinese scientists established a national Society of Tissue Engineering in 1999. In that same year, they held the first national conference on the topic in Shanghai.

Section 3

In 1997, plastic surgeon Cao Yilin, now one of China's leading tissue engineering researchers, made headlines when he was among a group of researchers in Boston to publish a paper in Plastic and Reconstructive Surgery on his team's success in growing a human ear—comprised of tissue-engineered cartilage made from a biodegradable polymer seeded with chondrocytes—on a mouse. Cao was based in the United States at the time, working with a prominent tissue engineer Joseph Vacanti at Massachusetts General Hospital, but he returned to China soon after. Others say his achievement helped prove the worth of the field to the Chinese government. In 2001, a government grant program targeting research with commercial potential—the 863 Program—started explicitly funding tissue engineering. From 2002 to 2005, it supported an initial 11 projects in the field, according to Cui. The program currently sponsors 48 projects, says Guo Quanyi, who oversees the 863 Program's tissue engineering grants. The boom in funding has been matched by a steep increase in the number of professors and assistant professors in China working on tissue engineering, Cui says, from roughly 100 in the 1990s to some 300 today.

Listening Exercises

Listen to each section twice, and as you are listening, (a) number the words or expressions in the list on the work sheet by order of their first appearance in the passage you are listening to; (b) check if your numbering is correct—if incorrect, listen to the section again; (c) orally answer the questions about the content of each section.

Unit 5, Section 1

applications	neuroregeneration	plaque
capitalize on	outfitted	somewhat
innovation	peripheral	testament

1. Why would it seem surprising that the Nantong laboratory has received several major grants?

2. What is the particular research specialization of the Nantong lab?

3. What is Dr. Cui Fuzhai specializing in?

Unit 5, Section 2

analysis	established	singled out
coming into its own	quintuple	stem cell
decades	release	various

1. What is Dr. Ma Zhun's research speciality?

Unit 5, Section 3

achievement	plastic surgeon	steep increase
cartilage	prominent	supported
chondrocytes	publish	targeting

1. What animal was used to grow a human ear?

2. From what medical establishment did Dr. Cao Yilin return to China?

3. What was the specialty that made Dr. Cao Yilin look into tissue engineering?

5.3   Writing: Title

由于只有少数人研读整篇论文，多数人只是浏览原始杂志或文摘、索引的论文题目。因此须慎重选择题目中的每一个字，力求做到长短适中、概括性强、重点突出、一目了然。

论文题目一般由名词词组或名词短语构成，应避免使用完整的陈述句。在必须使用动词的情况下，一般用分词或动名词形式。题目中间的介词、冠词通常情况下首字母小写。如果题目为直接问句，则要加问号；间接问句不用加问号。

论文题目写作要求

（1）题目要准确地反映论文的内容。作为论文的"标签"，题目既不能过于空泛和一般化，也不宜过于烦琐，否则不能给人留下鲜明的印象。为确保题目的含义准确，应尽量避免使用非定量的、含义不明的词，如 rapid、new 等；还要尽量做到用词具有专指性，如 a vanadium-iron alloy 明显优于 a magnetic alloy。

（2）题目用语要简练、明了，以最少的文字概括尽可能多的内容。题目最好不超过 12 个单词，或 100 个英文字符（含空格和标点）。题目如果能用一行文字表达，就尽量不要用两行（超过两行有可能会削弱读者的印象）。在题目内容层次很多的情况下，如果难以简化，最好采用主、副题名相结合的方法，主、副题名之间用冒号（:）隔开，如 *Importance of Replication in Microarray Gene Expression Studies: Statistical Methods and Evidence from Repetitive CDNA Hybridizations* (Proc Natl Acad Sci USA, 2000, 97(18): 9834~9839)。其中，副题名起补充、阐明作用，可起到很好的效果。

（3）题目要清晰地反映论文的具体内容和特色，明确表明研究工作的独到之处，力求简洁有效、重点突出。为了表达更加直接、清楚，以便引起读者的注意，应尽可能地将表达核心内容的主题词放在题名开头。如在 *The Effectiveness of Vaccination Against in Healthy,*

Working Adults (N Engl J Med, 1995, 333: 889-893)中，如果作者用关键词 vaccination 作为题名的开头，则读者可能会误认为这是一篇方法性的论文，即论文内容关于 how to vaccinate this population。相反，用 effectiveness 作为题名中第一个主题词，就直接指明了研究问题"Is vaccination in this population effective?"。题名中应慎重使用缩略语，尤其对于可有多个解释的缩略语，应严加限制，必要时应在括号中注明全称。对那些全称较长，缩写后已得到科技界公认的缩略语，才可在题名中使用。为方便二次检索，题名中应避免使用化学式、上下角标、特殊符号（数字符号、希腊字母等）、公式、不常用的专业术语和非英语词汇（包括拉丁语）等。

（4）由于题目比句子简短，且不需要主语、谓语、宾语，因此词序也就变得尤为重要。特别是如果词语间的修饰关系使用不当，就会影响读者正确理解题目的真实含意。例如，*Isolation of Antigens from Monkeys Using Complement-fixation Techniques*，可使人误解为"猴子使用了补体结合技术"。应改为：*Using Complement-fixation Techniques in Isolation of Antigens from Monkeys*，即"用补体结合技术从猴体分离抗体"。

Author(s)（作者姓名）

关于论文的署名如何决定这一问题，国际医学期刊编辑委员会（ICMJE）给出了作者资格的界定标准：

（1）参与课题的构思与设计，资料的分析和解释；

（2）参与文稿的写作或对其中重要学术内容做重大修改；

（3）参与最后定稿，并同意投稿和出版。

以上 3 项条件应全部具备方可成为作者；作者的排列顺序应由所有作者共同决定；每位作者都应该能够就论文的全部内容向公众负责。

通信作者（corresponding author）通常是实际统筹处理投稿和承担答复审稿意见等工作的主导者，也通常是稿件所涉及研究工作的负责人。通信作者的姓名多位于论文作者名单的最后（使用符号来标识说明是 corresponding author），但其贡献不亚于论文的第一作者。对于欧洲某些按姓名字顺排列作者署名的期刊来说，通信作者的标识就显得更重要。

通信作者标注：corresponding author, to whom correspondence should be addressed 或 the person to whom inquiries regarding the paper should be addressed。

如果两个以上的作者在地位上是相同的，可以采取"共同第一作者"（joint first author）的署名方式，并说明 these authors contributed equally to the work（这些作者对研究工作的贡献是相同的）。详情请参考 *Nature Guide to Authors*。

按照欧美国家的习惯，名字（first name）在前，姓氏（surname/family name/last name）在后。但我国人名地名标准规定，中国人名拼写均改用汉语拼音字母拼写，姓在前名在后。因此，若刊物无特殊要求，应按我国标准执行。如果论文由几个人撰写，则应逐一写出各自的姓名。作者与作者之间用空格或逗号隔开。例如，Liu Rong, Qi Liping。

Affiliation(s) and Address(es)（联系方式）

在作者姓名的下方还应注明作者的工作单位、邮政编码、电子邮件地址或联系电话等。这些信息应准确清楚，使读者能按所列信息顺利地与作者联系。例如，

School of Biomedical Engineering, Dalian University of Technology, Dalian 116024, P. R. China.

Email: lipingqi@dlut.edu.cn

也有刊物在论文标题页的页脚标出以上细节，在论文最后附上作者简介和照片。

5.4　Speaking: Conference Presentation—Examples

Opening Remarks（开场白）

1. Thank you very much, Prof. *** (Session Chair), for your very kind introduction. Good morning everyone! I consider it a great honor to be asked to speak about…on this session of our symposium.

2. Ladies and gentleman, good afternoon. It's an honor to have the opportunity to address such a distinguished audience.

3. Mr. Chairman, thank you very much for your kind introduction. President, Distinguished colleagues, ladies and gentleman, Good morning! It's an honor to have the opportunity to give my presentation here.

4. Good morning, everyone. I appreciate the opportunity to be with you today. I am here to talk to you about…

5. Good morning, everyone. I am very happy to have this chance to give my presentation. Before I start my speech, let me ask you a question. By a show of hands, how many of you own a car?

Reference to the Audience（与听众互动）

1. I can see many of you are from…department.

2. I know many of you are familiar with this topic. / You all look as though you've heard this before.

3. I understand that you've all traveled a long way. / After hours of conference, you must feel a little tired. Now I'd like you to see an interesting topic…

Background Information（背景介绍）

1. I would like to start by briefly reviewing the history of biomedical engineering.

2. I think it would be the best to start out by looking at a few slides.

3. I should like to preface my remarks with a description of the basic idea.

4. The first thing I would like to talk about is the definition of the terms I shall use in my lecture.

5. The first point I'd like to make is the historical background of the invention.

Unit 6   Biomechanics

6.1   Text: Biomechanics

Biomechanics combines engineering and the life sciences by applying principles from classical mechanics to the study of living systems. This relatively new field covers a broad range of topics, including strength of biological materials, biofluid mechanics in the cardiovascular and respiratory systems, material properties and interactions of medical implants and the body, heat and mass transfer into biological tissues (e.g., tumors), biocontrol systems regulating metabolism or voluntary motion, and kinematics and kinetics applied to study human gait. The great breadth of the field of biomechanics arises from the complexities and variety of biological organisms and systems.[1]

The study of biomechanics can take place on a range of scales and levels, from the molecular level of cell signaling to the study of entire organisms.[2] Understanding how organisms move is an important aspect of this field, as is the understanding of mechanical systems in the body such as the circulatory system and the digestive tract. While people may not think of living organisms as machines, in many ways, they actually perform a lot like machines, and the concepts used in basic mechanics can also be applied to the body.

One field of interest in biomechanics is the study of injuries. Sports injuries in particular are compelling to some researchers, with people interested in learning about how athletes at the peak of their performance move and injure themselves in addition to studying injuries in people who are not as athletic.[3] Biomechanics researchers also look at topics like how the loss of a limb can change movement patterns, how prosthetic devices can be better designed to move with the body, and how bodies respond to stress and strain ranging from depletion of bone mass in space to working as manual laborers.

On a clinical level, biomechanics is very important for understanding patterns of injury and for developing physical therapy programs which will increase strength.[4] Biomechanics is also the science behind many ergonomics recommendations for everyone from massage therapists to office workers. Understanding how activities like using a computer, sitting in an uncomfortable chair, or lifting heavy objects strain the body is an important first step in finding ways to help people reduce strain. Biomechanics is also used to show people how to use their bodies more efficiently, as in the case of a massage therapist who uses the pressure of elbows instead of just the hands.

Researchers are also interested in how different kinds of organisms move and function, and how these variations confer advantages. For example, fish and marine mammals swim in a variety of different ways, while plants have developed a variety of creative ways to access nutrients and resources such as sunlight.

◆*Source: https://www.wisegeek.com/what-is-biomechanics.htm.*

Glossary

biomechanics [ˌbaɪoməˈkænɪks]	*n.* 生物力学
cardiovascular [ˌkɑrdioˈvæskjələ]	*adj.* 心血管的
respiratory [rɪˈspɪrətəri]	*adj.* 呼吸的
implant [ˈɪmplɑːnt]	*n.* 移植物
tumor [ˈtjuːmə]	*n.* 肿瘤
metabolism [mɪˈtæbəlɪzəm]	*n.* 新陈代谢
kinematics [ˌkɪnɪˈmætɪks]	*n.* 运动学
kinetics [kɪˈnetɪks]	*n.* 动力学
compelling [kəmˈpelɪŋ]	*adj.* 引人注目的
ergonomics [ˌɜːgəˈnɒmɪks]	*n.* 人体工程学
therapist [ˈθerəpɪst]	*n.* 治疗学家

Technical Terms

biofluid mechanics	生物流体力学
voluntary motion	随意运动
cell signaling	细胞信号传导
circulatory system	循环系统
digestive tract	消化道
stress and strain	应力应变
bone mass	骨量
manual laborer	体力劳动者
physical therapy	物理治疗
massage therapist	按摩师

Notes

1. The great breadth of the field of biomechanics arises from the complexities and variety of biological organisms and systems.

生物力学的广泛领域源于生物有机体和系统的复杂性及多样性。

分析：句式 A of B of C of D 考查多个介宾短语作后置定语的翻译技巧。of 一般表示从属关系，即"……的"，因而在翻译时一般采用倒序翻译。

2. The study of biomechanics can take place on a range of scales and levels, from the molecular level of cell signaling to the study of entire organisms.

生物力学的研究可以在一定范围和尺度上进行，从细胞信号传导的分子视角到整个生物体的研究。

分析：from...to...表示"从……至……，从……到……"。

3. Sports injuries in particular are compelling to some researchers, with people interested in learning about how athletes at the peak of their performance move and injure themselves in addition to studying injuries in people who are not as athletic.

一些研究人员对运动损伤尤其感兴趣，除了研究非运动员的损伤，他们更想了解运动员是如何发挥人体最大潜能，并且在达到极限时怎么受到伤害的。

分析：with 的特殊用法，表示原因或理由。

4. On a clinical level, biomechanics is very important for understanding patterns of injury and for developing physical therapy programs which will increase strength.

在临床上，生物力学对于理解损伤模式和发展物理治疗方案以增加力量是非常重要的。

分析：本句中 which 作为非限定性定语从句的代词，指代 physical therapy programs。

Translation Skills：词类的转换

汉语和英语属于不同的语系，二者在很多方面存在区别，如语法和词法。为了让专业英语译文既贴切原文又通俗易懂，应掌握一些翻译技巧，词类的转换就是其中之一。词类表征了词的属类，如动词、名词、副词等。词类的转换是指将英语语言中的某一类词转译为汉语中的另一类词，如将英语中的名词译成汉语中的动词，将英语中的动词译成汉语中的副词等。本节旨在帮助读者灵活运用词类转换这一翻译技巧，逐步提高翻译能力，使翻译的句子更加准确通顺。

1. 名词的转换

（1）名词转换为动词：在每个英语句子中只能有一个真正的谓语，通常为动词，所以英语中名词用得多一些；而在汉语中一个句子可以使用多个动词或动词词组，名词往往只有一个。在英译汉时，若将名词逐一翻译，译文往往不符合汉语的表达习惯。如果将英语中的名词转换为汉语中的动词，则更符合汉语的表达习惯。

🍃**例句**

China's first atomic <u>blast</u> in October 1964 was a great shock by the world.
1964 年 10 月中国第一颗原子弹<u>爆炸</u>成功，使全球为之震惊。

Surface Characterization <u>using</u> an optical profiler…
<u>使用</u>光学轮廓仪观察到的表面特征……

（2）名词转换为形容词：英语中由形容词派生成的名词在翻译时可转换为形容词。

🍃**例句**

Single crystals of high perfection are an absolute <u>necessity</u> for the fabrication of integrated circuits.
高度完整的单晶对于制造集成电路来说是绝对<u>必要的</u>。

（3）一些英语名词（短语）还可以转换为副词。

🍃**例句**

He had <u>the honor</u> to attend this international conference.

他<u>荣幸地</u>参加了这次国际会议。

2. 动词的转换

有些动词在翻译成汉语时很难找到相应的动词，这时可将其翻译成名词。

例句

Single-chip microcomputer is mainly <u>characterized</u> by its small size and powerful function.
单片机的主要<u>特点</u>是体积小、功能强大。

3. 形容词的转换

（1）形容词转换为动词：英语中的形容词除了修饰名词，还常常和系动词一起构成系表结构，其后通过介词接宾语，在翻译时通常把这类形容词转换成动词，以表示各种状态、直觉、感觉、态度等。

equal to	等于，胜任	relative to	和……有关
good at	擅长于	free from	免于，免除

例句

The wax is <u>present</u> in crystalline tubules.
蜡<u>存在</u>于晶体管中。

（2）形容词转换为名词：这种情况也是较为常见的，有的形容词可完全转换为名词并具有名词的一切语法特征。

例句

The <u>unavoidable</u> happened in the end.
<u>不可避免的事</u>终于发生了。

（3）形容词转换为副词：上文提到，一些英语名词在翻译时要转换成动词。相应地，修饰这些名词的形容词也要转换成副词。

例句

A <u>continuous</u> increase in the temperature of a gas confined in a container will lead to a <u>continuous</u> increase in the internal pressure within the gas.
<u>不断地</u>增加容器内的气体温度，相应地会使气体的压力<u>不断地</u>增大。

4. 副词的转换

（1）副词转换为动词：英语中有一些作表语的副词或复合宾语中的副词，翻译时可以转换成动词。

例句

He opened the lid to let oxygen <u>in</u>.
他把盖子打开，让氧气<u>进来</u>。

（2）副词转换为名词：通常，由名词转换而来的副词在译成汉语时，为了达到语句通顺的目的，也可转换成名词。

例句

Researchers in the late 1960s discovered that humans are born with the capacity to approach challenges in four primary ways: <u>analytically, procedurally, relationally (or collaboratively) and innovatively.</u>

20 世纪 60 年代末，研究人员发现人类天生具有能力通过四种主要方法来应对挑战，即<u>分析法、流程法、关联法（或合作法）、创新法</u>。

（3）副词转换为形容词：由形容词派生而来的副词根据需要可转换为形容词。

例句

Clinical testing of the Salk polio vaccine, in which millions of doses were administered to children, could not happen without the engineering methods to <u>cheaply</u> produce the vaccine in large quantity.

如果没有<u>廉价</u>的大量生产疫苗的工程方法，就不可能进行索尔克脊髓灰质炎疫苗的临床实验。在临床实验中，儿童接种了数百万剂该疫苗。

5. 其他的词类转换

其他词类转换主要包括介词的转换、连词的转换、冠词的转换等。

例句

The quantitative measurement of friction force was calibrated <u>by</u> the method described by B hus han (2011).

摩擦力定量测量可以<u>采用</u>B hus han（2011）描述的方法进行校准。

6.2　Listening: Biomechanics

🎧 Section 1

Biomechanics is the study of the structure and function of the mechanical aspects of biological systems, at any level from whole organisms to organs, cells and cell organelles, using the methods of mechanics. Biomechanics is closely related to engineering, because it often uses traditional engineering sciences to analyze biological systems. Some simple applications of Newtonian mechanics and/or materials sciences can supply correct approximations to the mechanics of many biological systems. Applied mechanics, most notably mechanical engineering disciplines such as continuum mechanics, mechanism analysis, structural analysis, kinematics and dynamics play prominent roles in the study of biomechanics. Usually biological systems are much more complex than man-built systems. Numerical methods are hence applied in almost every biomechanical study. Research is done in an iterative process of hypothesis and verification, including several steps of modeling, computer simulation and experimental measurements.

🎧 Section 2

The study of biomechanics ranges from the inner workings of a cell to the movement and development of limbs, to the mechanical properties of soft tissue, and bones. Some simple examples of biomechanics research include the investigation of the forces that act on limbs, the aerodynamics of bird and insect flight, the hydrodynamics of swimming in fish, and locomotion in general across all forms of life, from individual cells to whole organisms. With growing understanding of the physiological behavior of living tissues, researchers are able to advance the field of tissue engineering, as well as develop improved treatments for a wide array of pathologies.

Biomechanics is also applied to studying human musculoskeletal systems. Such research utilizes force platforms to study human ground reaction forces and infrared videography to capture the trajectories of markers attached to the human body to study human 3D motion. Research also applies electromyography to study muscle activation, investing muscle responses to external forces and perturbations.

Biomechanics is widely used in orthopedic industry to design orthopedic implants for human joints, dental parts, external fixations and other medical purposes. Biotribology is a very important part of it. It is a study of the performance and function of biomaterials used for orthopedic implants. It plays a vital role to improve the design and produce successful biomaterials for medical and clinical purposes. One such example is in tissue engineered cartilage.

Section 3

In sports biomechanics, the laws of mechanics are applied to human movement in order to gain a greater understanding of athletic performance and to reduce sport injuries as well. It focuses on the application of the scientific principles of mechanical physics to understand movements of action of human bodies and sports implements such as cricket bat, hockey stick and javelin etc. Elements of mechanical engineering (e.g., strain gauges), electrical engineering (e.g., digital filtering), computer science (e.g., numerical methods), gait analysis (e.g., force platforms), and clinical neurophysiology (e.g., surface EMG) are common methods used in sports biomechanics.

Biomechanics in sports can be stated as the muscular, joint and skeletal actions of the body during the execution of a given task, skill and/or technique. Proper understanding of biomechanics relating to sports skill has the greatest implications on: sport's performance, rehabilitation and injury prevention, along with sport mastery. As noted by Doctor Michael Yessis, one could say that the best athlete is the one that executes his or her skill the best.

◆ *Source: https://en.wikipedia.org/wiki/Biomechanics.*

Listening Exercises

Listen to each section twice, and as you are listening, (a) number the words or expressions in the list on the work sheet by order of their first appearance in the passage you are listening to; (b) check if your numbering is correct—if incorrect, listen to the section again; (c) orally answer the questions about the content of each section.

Unit 6, Section 1

almost	continuum	modeling
approximations	kinematics	organelles
aspects	man-built	related to

1. What is the difference between an organ and an organelle? And give three examples of organs.

2. What disciplines of mechanics are important in biomechanics?

3. What are the steps to be followed in biomechanical research?

Unit 6, Section 2

array	implants	perturbations
cartilage	organisms	ranges
electromyography	orthopedic	soft tissue

1. Name three applications of biomechanical engineering.

2. How can the movements of the human body be studied?

3. How does the orthopaedic industry make use of biomechanics?

Unit 6, Section 3

athlete	implications	reduce
executes	mechanics	stated
gauges	neurophysiology	understand

1. Name one of the reasons why biomechanical engineering is important in sports biomechanics.

2. Name three methods that are common in sports biomechanics.

3. How does the study of biomechanics benefit individual athletes?

6.3　Writing: Abstract

摘要也称为内容提要，是对论文的内容不加注释和评论的简短陈述，其作用主要是为读者阅读、信息检索提供方便。

摘要不宜太详尽，也不宜太简短，应将论文的研究体系、主要方法、重要发现、主要结论等简明扼要地加以概括。

摘要的构成要素

研究目的——准确描述该研究的目的，说明提出问题的缘由，表明研究的范围和重要性。

研究方法——简要说明研究课题的基本设计，结论是如何得到的。

结果——简要列出该研究的主要结果及新发现，说明其价值和局限性。叙述要具体、准确，并给出结果的置信值。

结论——简要地说明经验，论证取得的正确观点及理论价值或应用价值，是否还有与此有关的其他问题有待进一步研究，是否可推广应用等。

摘要的基本类型

摘要主要有两大类：资料性摘要（informative abstract）和说明性摘要（descriptive abstract）。一般刊物论文所附摘要都属于这两类。还有一种为二者的结合，称为结合型摘要。另有一种结构型摘要，遵循一定的格式和套路，更加便于计算机检索。

资料性摘要——适用于专题研究型论文和实验报告型论文。资料性摘要应尽量完整和准确地体现原文的具体内容，特别指出研究的方法、结果和结论等。这类摘要大体按介绍背景、实验方法和过程、结果与讨论的格式来写。

说明性摘要——只向读者指出论文的主要议题是什么，不涉及具体的研究方法和结果。说明性摘要一般适用于综述性论文，也用于讨论、评论性论文，尤以介绍某学科近期发展动态的论文居多。

结合型摘要——以上两种摘要的综合，其特点是对原文需突出强调的部分做具体的叙述；对于较复杂，无法三言两语概括的部分则采用一般性的描述。

结构型摘要——随着信息科学和电子出版物的发展，近年来又出现了一种新的摘要形式，即结构型摘要。这类摘要先用短语归纳要点，再用句子加以简明扼要地说明，便于模仿和套用，能规范具体地将内容表达出来，方便审稿，便于计算机检索。

摘要的撰写要求

（1）确保客观而充分地表述论文的内容，适当强调研究中的创新、重要之处（但不要使用评价性文字）；尽量包括论文中的主要论点和重要细节（重要的论证或数据）。

（2）要求结构严谨，语义确切，表述简明，一般不分段落；表述要注意逻辑性，尽量使用指示性的词语来表达论文的不同部分（层次），如使用 we found that...表示结果，使用 we suggest that...表示讨论结果的含义等。

（3）排除在本学科领域已成为常识的或科普知识的内容；尽量避免引用文献，若无法回避使用引文，应在引文出现的位置将引文的书目信息标注在方括号内；不使用非本专业的读者难以理解的缩略语、简称、代号，若确有需要（如避免多次重复较长的术语）使用非同行熟知的缩写符号，应在缩写符号第一次出现时给出其全称；不使用一次文献中列出的章节号、图号、表号、公式号及参考文献号。

（4）要求使用法定计量单位，正确地书写规范字和标点符号；众所周知的国家、机构、专用术语尽可能用简称或缩写；为方便检索系统转录，应尽量避免使用图、表、化学结构式、数学表达式、角标或希腊文等特殊符号。

（5）摘要的长度：ISO 规定，大多数实验研究性论文，字数为 1000～5000 字的，其摘要长度限于 100～250 个英文单词。

（6）摘要的时态：摘要所采用的时态因情况而定，应力求表达自然、妥当。在写作中可大致遵循以下原则。①在介绍背景资料时，如果句子的内容是不受时间影响的普遍事实，应使用一般现在时；如果句子的内容为对某种研究趋势的概述，则使用现在完成时。②在叙述研究目的或主要研究活动时，如果采用"论文导向"，多使用一般现在时（如 this paper presents...）；如果采用"研究导向"，则使用一般过去时（如 this study investigated...）。③概述实验程序、方法和主要结果时，通常用一般现在时（如 we describe a new molecular approach to analyzing...）。

④叙述结论或建议时，可使用一般现在时、臆测动词或 may、should、could 等助动词（如 we suggest that climate instability in the early part of the last interglacial may have...）。

（7）摘要的人称和语态：作为一种可阅读和检索的独立使用的文体，摘要一般只用第三人称而不用其他人称来写。有的摘要出现了"我们""作者"作为陈述的主语，这会减弱摘要表述的客观性，有时也会出现逻辑不通的现象。由于主动语态的表达更为准确，且更易阅读，因而目前大多数期刊都提倡使用主动语态，国际知名科技期刊 *Nature*、*Cell* 等尤其如此。

Keywords（关键词）

关键词是为了满足文献标引或检索工作的需要而从论文中提取出的词或词组。国际标准和我国标准均要求论文摘要后标引 3～8 个关键词。关键词既可以作为文献检索或分类的标识，它本身又是论文主题的浓缩。读者从中可以判断论文的主题、研究方向、方法等。关键词包括主题词和自由词两类：主题词是专门为文献的标引或检索而从自然语言的主要词汇中挑选出来，并规范化了的词或词组；自由词则是未规范的即还未收入主题词表中的词或词组。关键词以名词或名词短语居多。如果使用缩略词，则应使用公认和普遍使用的缩略语，如 IP、CAD、CPU 等；否则应写出全称，其后用括号标出其缩略语形式。

6.4　Speaking: Conference Presentation—Examples

Main Topic（主题）

(1) I would like to concentrate on the problem of antibiotic abuse in hospitals.

(2) I want to confine my talk to the latest developments in civil engineering.

(3) My report today will deal with the observation of supernova.

(4) In my presentation this morning, I'll limit myself to three major points only.

(5) Now, I would like to address myself to the most important aspect of this problem.

Shifting to the Next Main Point（主题之间的过渡）

(1) Well, let's move on to the next point.

(2) We will now come to the second problem.

(3) Turning to the next question, I'll talk about the stages of the procedure.

(4) As the second topic, I shall stop here. Now let's turn our attention to the third topic.

(5) So much for the methodology of our experiment. Now I would like to shift to the discussion of the results.

(6) Now, let's move away from the first part and switch over to the next part of my presentation.

(7) That's all for the introduction and now we can go on to the literature review.

(8) Next, I would like to turn to a more difficult problem.

(9) The next point I'd like to talk about is the feasibility of this project.

(10) That brings me to my second point.

Unit 7   Rehabilitation Engineering

7.1   Text: Rehabilitation Engineering

Rehabilitation Engineering is a nascent and developing field compared to most other engineering disciplines, yet there is compelling evidence that the practice of rehabilitation engineering has its roots in antiquity.[1] Examples include use of a "stick" as an aid for ambulation, the attachment of wheels to a chair and many other implementations to compensate for functional deficits. The utilization of a pole as a walking aid appears in an Egyptian stele in the Carlsberg Sculpture Museum (Copenhagen) that dates to 1500 BC. This same simple appliance may be observed in use in developing countries today. While prosthetics is often viewed as separate and distinct from rehabilitation engineering—perhaps most prominently by prosthetists—it is an obvious and natural subset of the larger concept of rehabilitation engineering.

Historically, warfare has provided a stimulus for advances in rehabilitation engineering, and it is not surprising to learn that medieval armorers as the first prosthetists were also the first rehabilitation engineers.[2] The modern era of rehabilitation engineering began with the establishment of "Rehabilitation Engineering Centers" (RECs) with support from the Federal Government through SRS in the early 1970s. Research and development was the dominant focus for rehabilitation engineering during the decade of the 1970s and resulted in the formation of RESNA, the Rehabilitation Engineering Society of North America in 1980. While R&D has continued as a major part of the rehabilitation field, an increased emphasis on the delivery of services began to emerge in the mid-1980s. By the mid 1990s service delivery had emerged as the major emphasis for both RESNA and for the field.[3] Formal training programs in rehabilitation engineering and assistive technology were being offered at major universities. To date most of these training programs are attached to more traditional academic and professional training departments.

The future of rehabilitation engineering and assistive technology (AT) will depend on understanding and documenting the confluence of two critical factors represented by the paradigm of "functionality". This confluence is of medical restoration and consumer participation. Historically, medicine has attempted to "fix" or intervene on the injury or disease plateau, and the consumer simply "carried on". Now, the International Classification of Function (ICF) has elevated therapy or technology to more strongly match the desired activity and participation of the consumer. Means of quantifying or qualifying participation are yet to be agreed upon, and so rehabilitation professionals are aspiring to harness their science toward this challenge.

Just as rehabilitation engineering cannot be done effectively in isolation from scientists and other clinicians connected with end users, social scientists investigating new technological directions need to be working effectively with engineers. The goal of rehabilitation engineering must be to support the concept of self-determination for older adults and people with disabilities. Success in the development of AT requires technical competence and imagination, but equally or even more importantly, it depends on a thorough appreciation and understanding of aging, older adults, disabilities, people with disabilities, environment, costs, regulations, policies, and other limiting factors.[4] Some otherwise remarkable engineering accomplishments have been dismal failures because of lack of awareness and appreciation of limitations posed by these factors. We believe that a unique blend of complementary talent and experience that combines the best in engineering, science, and technology with consummate understanding and appreciation of the relevance of social, cultural, behavioral, regulatory, and economic and environmental dimensions and considerations is essential to address the burgeoning issues of aging and disability.

◆ *Source: An Introduction to Rehabilitation Engineering.*

Glossary

nascent ['næsənt]	*adj.* 初期的
antiquity [æn'tɪkwɪti]	*n.* 古代
medieval [ˌmedi'iːvəl]	*adj.* 中古的，中世纪的
armorer ['ɑːmərə]	*n.* 兵器制造者，军械修护员
emerge [ɪ'mɜːdʒ]	*vi.* 浮现
assistive [ə'sɪstɪv]	*adj.* 辅助的
confluence ['kɒnfluəns]	*n.* 汇流；汇流处
plateau ['plætəʊ]	*n.* 平稳时期，稳定水平
dismal ['dɪzməl]	*adj.* 惨淡的，凄凉的
blend [blend]	*n.* 混合物
burgeoning ['bɜːdʒənɪŋ]	*adj.* 迅速发展的

Technical Terms

rehabilitation engineering	康复工程
compensate for	补偿损失
functional deficit	功能缺陷
walking aid	助行器
assistive technology	辅助技术

Notes

1. Rehabilitation Engineering is a nascent and developing field compared to most other engineering disciplines, yet there is compelling evidence that the practice of rehabilitation engineering has its roots in antiquity.

与大多数其他工程学科相比，康复工程是一个新兴且正在发展的领域，然而证据表明，康复工程的实践起源于古代。

分析：that 作连词引导同位语从句，是对前面名词 evidence 的具体内容所做的详细阐述。

2. Historically, warfare has provided a stimulus for advances in rehabilitation engineering, and it is not surprising to learn that medieval armorers as the first prosthetists were also the first rehabilitation engineers.

根据历史事实，战争对康复工程的发展起了激励作用，因此，中世纪装甲师即是最早的修复师，也是最早的康复工程师。

分析：historically 是副词充当状语，用来修饰整个句子，被称为评注性状语。as the first prosthetists 中 as 为介词，意为"作为"。

3. By the mid 1990s service delivery had emerged as the major emphasis for both RESNA and for the field.

到 19 世纪 90 年代中期，提供服务已成为康复协会和康复领域的工作重点。

分析：by + 时间与动作性强的动词连用时，主句多用完成时。by 后的时间可指现在、过去或将来的时间点。

4. Success in the development of AT requires technical competence and imagination, but equally or even more importantly, it depends on a thorough appreciation and understanding of aging, older adults, disabilities, people with disabilities, environment, costs, regulations, policies, and other limiting factors.

AT 的成功发展需要技术能力和想象力，但同样或更重要的是，它取决于对衰老、老年人、残疾、残疾人、环境、成本、法规、政策和其他限制因素的深入了解和理解。

分析：but equally or even more importantly 作插入语，意为"但同样或更重要的是"。

Translation Skills：常用词组与结构

英语词组是英语词汇中最有生命力的部分。同一词组，在不同的意境、不同的句法中，意思也会有所不同。但是，有一些英语词组仍有其较固定的表达和翻译，掌握常用词组的表达和用法对提高我们阅读科技文献的能力是很重要的。

1. 常用介词的固定搭配

（1）to 的固定搭配

point to	指向……
belong to	属于……
write to	给……写信
lead to	导致
get down to	开始做……
up to	达到
refer to	提到；查阅
be used to	习惯于……
apply to	适用于
give oneself to	专心致力于
object to	反对

（2）in 的固定搭配

in a word	总之
in a way	有点，几分
in a walk	轻而易举地
in the air	在流行中，在传播中
in charge of	主管，负责
in the event of	万一，如果发生
in force	有效，实施中
get in	插话
check in	登记，报到
give in	屈服
find oneself in	处于某种地位或状态
join in	参加
stay in	待在家里（不外出）
drop in	落进，拜访

（3）for 的固定搭配

look for	寻找
call for	去叫（某人）
send for	派人去请
search for	搜寻
stand for	代表，支持
go in for	从事，追求
die for	渴望
trade for	交换
for short	简称
for frcc	免费
for good	永远
for the time being	暂时
be for	赞成
run for	竞选
fix a time for	为……定时间

2. 固定的搭配关系

一些固定的搭配关系会经常出现在句子中，需多观察、总结。

（1）某些名词必须与特定的动词连用

improve the equality	提高质量
come to the top	名列前茅
raise price	提升价格
make progress	进步

draw a conclusion	得出结论
draw lessons	取得教训
raise the efficiency	提高效率
improve the ability	提升能力
enhance one's vigilance	提高警惕
reach a complete agreement of views	取得一致意见
obtain the consent	取得同意

（2）某些名词必须与特定的介词搭配

in all directions	四面八方
a report on	关于……的报道
a skill in	在某方面的技能
a desire for	对……的渴望
advantage over	优于
connection with	联系

3．常见的固定结构

（1）在对概念或术语下定义时，常用词组 (can) be defined as 表示"是"或"被称为，被定义为"的意思，其结构可以是：概念（或术语）＋be 或 (can) be defined as ＋名词。

例句

Energy <u>is</u> usually <u>defined as</u> the ability to do work.
能量通常定义为做功的能力。

A computer <u>is</u> a machine that processes data into information.
计算机是一种将数据处理为信息的机器。

These laws <u>are defined as</u> Newton's laws of motion.
这些定律被定义为牛顿运动定律。

（2）在科技论文中，有时对概念或术语不必给出严格的定义，当只需从某种角度给予解释时，常用的词或短语是：mean，by…we mean，in other words，be termed，be called，be named，be consider as，be known as，refer to…as…，be regarded as，be thought of 等。

①　be called　被称为

例句

This flow of electrons driven through a conductor <u>is called</u> an electric current.
这种被驱动通过导体的电子流<u>被称为</u>电流。

②　by… we mean　所谓……是指

例句

<u>By memory, we mean</u> the internal storage locations of a computer.
<u>所谓存储器是指</u>计算机内部的存储单元。

③ refer to… as…   把……称作（称……为……）

🍃例句

We often <u>referred to</u> these rays as radiant matter.
我们过去常<u>称</u>这些射线<u>为</u>放射性物质。

④ be regarded as   被认为（看作）是

🍃例句

Radio waves <u>are regarded as</u> radiant energy.
无线电波<u>被认为是</u>辐射能。

⑤ be termed（＝be named; be called）   被称为

🍃例句

The ability of a capacitor to store electrical energy <u>is termed</u> capacitance.
电容器储存电能的能力<u>被称为</u>电容。

（3）在科技论文中，"主语＋be 形容词＋to 名词"的结构是很常见的，它用于对某一事物、概念或论点加以定论、叙述。

① be necessary（essential）to   对……是必要的，是……所必需的

🍃例句

Water <u>is necessary to</u> our life.
水<u>是</u>生命<u>所必需</u>的物质。

② be oppose to…   与……相反

🍃例句

The directions of the two forces <u>are opposite to</u> each other.
这两个力的方向<u>相反</u>。

③ be parallel to…   平行于……，与……平行

🍃例句

These lines <u>are parallel to</u> each other.
这些线相互<u>平行</u>。

④ be sensitive to…   对……是敏感的

🍃例句

The film <u>is sensitive to</u> light.
胶片<u>易感光</u>。

⑤ 表示"对……适应，适用于……"之意

be acceptable to   be applicable to   be adaptable to   be appropriate to

例句

A living thing is adaptable to a special environment.
生物与特定环境相适应。

The formula for kinetic energy is applicable to any object that is moving.
动能公式可适用于任何运动的物体。

⑥ 表示"与……相似（近似），等于，相当于"之意

be analogous to　be akin to　be approximate to
be similar to　be similar in　be corresponding to
be equal to　be equivalent to

例句

A computer is similar to the human brain.
计算机与人类的大脑类似。

Zero o'clock Greenwich Mean Time (GMY) is corresponding to eight o'clock Beijing time.
格林尼治标准时间零点相当于北京时间八点。

The amount of work is equal to the product of the force by the distance.
功的大小等于力乘以距离。

⑦ 表示"对……是重要的，对……是必要的（基本的）"等之意

be essential to…　be fundamental to...　be important to...
be indispensable to...　be necessary to...

例句

A knowledge of the various kinds of meters is essential to understanding and performing tests and measurements.
有关各种仪表的知识对于了解和进行各种测试是必不可少的。

This is fundamental to the building up China's national defence.
这对于中国的国防建设是必不可少的。

⑧ 表示"是……所特有的"之意

be particular to　be peculiar to　be proper to

例句

Tools are proper to mankind.　工具是人类特有的。
This mineral is particular to this region.　这种矿物是该地区所特有的。
Language is peculiar to mankind.　语言是人类特有的。

（4）在科技论文中，主语＋be＋不同的词/结构，有其约定成俗的翻译方式且使用频繁，在翻译时要特别注意。

① be（或其他系动词）＋adj.＋of＋名词或动名词
该结构的翻译可直接取形容词的含意。

例句

We <u>are short of</u> office equipment.
我们<u>缺乏</u>办公设备。

Computers <u>are capable of</u> doing extremely complicated work in all branches of learning.
计算机<u>能</u>在所有学习领域进行复杂的工作。

② be of+某些抽象名词

该结构的基本意思是"具有……"，但在翻译时应灵活运用。

例句

Electric current <u>are of</u> two kinds : DC and AC.
电流<u>有</u>两种：直流与交流。

The ships investigated by them <u>were of full form and low power</u>.
他们研究的船<u>线形完美，动力小</u>。

注意：有时把"of+名词"结构提到句首，起强调或承上启下的作用。

例句

<u>Of great importance</u> is to make careful records in many cases.
在许多场合下，仔细记录是<u>十分重要的</u>。

③ be（或其他动词）out of+名词

该结构有多种译法。

a）当谓语是静态动词时，该结构表示主语的状态。翻译时取 out of 的原意，即"在……之外"。

例句

The power plants are <u>out of</u> town.
这些发电厂<u>在</u>城<u>外</u>。

Fish cannot live <u>out of</u> water.
鱼儿<u>离开</u>水就不能生存。

b）当谓语是动态动词时，表示主语的动作方式。翻译时要灵活运用。

■ 表示"从……里，从……当中"之意。

例句

<u>Pump</u> as much air as possible <u>out of</u> the container.
尽可能地把容器内的空气都<u>抽走</u>。

■ 表示"解除，脱离，没有，缺乏"之意。

例句

The book is <u>out of print</u>.
这本书<u>绝版</u>了。

The school in the mountain village was <u>out of</u> teaching equipment.
这所山村学校<u>缺少</u>教学仪器。

■ 表示来源和动机之意。

例句

He asked the question merely <u>out of</u> curiosity.

她问这个问题只是<u>出于</u>好奇。

He <u>made</u> this table <u>out of</u> an old box.

她用一个旧木箱<u>做成了</u>一张桌子。

c）from + out of +多词

在掌握该结构的意义时，应首先把"out of +名词"理解为"……外"并作为一个整体概念来看待，然后再套上 from（从）的意思即可。

例句

We should <u>remove</u> the device <u>from out of</u> the room at once.

我们应该立即<u>搬走室外</u>的那个装置。

He is <u>from out of city</u>.

他<u>来自城外</u>。

上述例句说明英语词组具有同一词组含有多种意思的特点。在翻译时，要结合上下文的意思、逻辑关系、专业知识，从词组的基本意义出发，在忠实于原句、原文的原则下，进一步引申词组的意义，才能使我们的翻译达到准确的标准。

7.2　Listening: Rehabilitation Engineering

🎧 Section 1

Rehabilitation engineering is the systematic application of engineering sciences to design, develop, adapt, test, evaluate, apply, and distribute technological solutions to problems confronted by individuals with disabilities. These individuals may have experienced brain trauma caused from things such as PTSD, shock, near death experiences, drug induced brain alterations, panic anxiety, or other chemical imbalances. Functional areas addressed through rehabilitation engineering may include mobility, communications, hearing, vision, cognition, and activities associated with employment, independent living, education, and integration into the community.

Physical medicine and rehabilitation, also known as physiatry, is a branch of medicine that aims to enhance and restore functional ability and quality of life to those with physical impairments or disabilities. A physician having completed training in this field may be referred to as a physiatrist. Physiatrists specialize in restoring optimal function to people with injuries to the muscles, bones, ligaments, or nervous system.

In the hospital setting, physiatrists commonly treat patients who have had an amputation, spinal cord injury, stroke, traumatic brain injury, and other debilitating injuries. In treating these patients, physiatrists lead an interdisciplinary team of physical, occupational, recreational and speech therapists, nurses, psychologists, and social workers. In outpatient settings, physiatrists also treat patients with muscle and joint injuries, pain syndromes, non-healing wounds, and other disabling conditions. Physiatrists are trained to perform intramuscular and interarticular injections as well as nerve conduction studies.

🎧 Section 2

The major concern that physical medicine and rehabilitation addresses is the ability of a person to function optimally within the limitations placed upon them by a disabling impairment or disease process for which there is no known cure. The emphasis is not on the full restoration to the premorbid level of function, but rather the optimization of the quality of life for those not able to achieve full restoration. A team approach to chronic conditions is emphasized to coordinate care of patients. Comprehensive rehabilitation is provided by specialists in this field, who act as facilitators, team leaders, and medical experts for rehabilitation.

In rehabilitation, goal setting is often used by the clinical care team to provide the team and the person undergoing rehabilitation for an acquired disability a direction to work towards. Very low quality evidence indicates that goal setting may lead to a higher quality of life for the person with the disability, and it is not clear if goal setting used in this context reduces or increases re-hospitalization or death.

🎧 Section 3

Specifics of training differs from program to program but the base knowledge acquired is roughly the same. Residents are trained in the inpatient setting to take care of multiple types of rehabilitation including: spinal cord injury, traumatic brain injury, stroke, orthopedic, cancer, cerebral palsy, burn, pediatric rehab, and other disabling injuries. The residents are also trained in the outpatient setting to know how to take care of the chronic conditions patients have following their inpatient stay. During training, residents are instructed on how to properly perform several diagnostic procedures which include electromyography and nerve conduction studies and also procedures such as joint injections and trigger point injections.

◆ *Source: https://en.wikipedia.org/wiki/Rehabilitation_engineering.*

Listening Exercises

Listen to each section twice, and as you are listening, (a) number the words or expressions in the list on the work sheet by order of their first appearance in the passage you are listening to; (b) check if your numbering is correct—if incorrect, listen to the section again; (c) orally answer the questions about the content of each section.

Unit 7, Section 1

adapt	design	physiatrist
amputation	interarticular	recreational
cognition	joint	trauma

1. Name three things that can cause a brain trauma.

2. How do physiatrists help their patients?

3. What specialists could belong to a team led by a physiatrist?

Unit 7, Section 2

ability	impairment	quality of life
facilitators	optimization	re-hospitalization
goal setting	premorbid	towards

1. What kind of medical conditions does a rehabilitation engineer endeavour to control or improve in general?

2. What can a rehabilitation engineer not always expect to achieve?

3. Who needs to set the goals for the rehabilitation of a patient?

Unit 7, Section 3

acquired	instructed	pediatric
chronic condition	outpatient	spinal cord injury
inpatient	palsy	trigger point

1. Name three cases where inpatients may require the work of rehabilitation engineers.

2. What help do outpatients receive from rehabilitation engineers?

7.3   Writing: Introduction

引言位于正文的起始部分，主要叙述写作的目的或研究的宗旨，使读者了解和评估研究成果。引言的主要内容包括：介绍相关研究的背景、进展；说明自己对已有研究的看法，以往工作的不足之处，以及自己所做研究的创新性或重要价值；说明研究中要解决的问题，所采取的方法，必要时需说明采用某种方法的理由；介绍论文的主要结果和结构安排。

写作步骤

一般而言，引言的写作通常包括四个基本的步骤。

步骤一：背景资料。在引言开头部分，首先介绍论文的研究领域，提出有关该研究领域的一般信息，并针对论文将要探讨的问题或现象提供背景知识。

步骤二：文献回顾。接下来，讨论其他学者对于此问题或现象曾经发表的相关研究。

步骤三：指出问题。指出仍然有某个问题或现象值得进一步研究。

步骤四：研究目的。最后，描述自己的研究活动，并叙述该研究活动的具体目的。

写作要求

1. 尽量准确、清楚且简洁地指出所探讨问题的本质和范围，对研究背景的阐述做到繁简适度。

2．解释或定义专用术语或缩写词，以帮助编辑、审稿人和读者阅读稿件。

3．在背景介绍和问题的提出部分，应引用"最相关"的文献以指引读者。优先选择引用的文献包括相关研究中的经典的、重要的和最具说服力的文献。不要刻意回避引用"最重要"的相关文献（甚至是对作者研究具某种"启示性"意义的文献），不要不恰当地大量引用作者本人的文献。此外，只需引述适当的参考文献以指出自己研究工作的意义、动机及目的，并说明研究能提供一些新的资料或解决某个需要解决的问题，不需要旁征博引，证明作者见闻广博。

4．说明自己研究工作的背景及动机，既要表示自己对同一研究领域里其他学者曾发表的相关研究十分熟悉，也要反映自己的研究工作和这些学者过去的研究工作之间的关系。常见的错误是论文中缺少对相关研究的引述，因而无法清楚地说明研究的动机及重要性。应先清楚地解释自己研究领域的近况，让审稿人和读者看出本研究结果对所涉研究领域所做的贡献。采取适当的方式强调作者在本次研究中最重要的发现或贡献，让读者顺着逻辑的演进阅读论文。

5．指出研究问题：①以前的学者处理得不够完善或尚未研究的重要课题；②过去的研究所派生并值得探讨的新问题；③以前的学者曾经提出两个或两个以上互不相容的观点或理论，为了解决这些存在差异的观点或理论之间的冲突，必须开展进一步的研究；④过去的研究自然可以扩展到的新领域或新题目，或者以前曾提出的方法或技术可得到改善或延伸到新的应用范围。

6．叙述作者自己的研究性质与目的，以说明如何解决所提出的研究问题。适当地使用 I、we 或 our 以明确地指示作者本人的工作，如最好使用 we conducted this study to determine whether...，而不使用 this study was conducted to determine whether...。叙述前人工作的欠缺以强调自己研究的创新时，应慎重且留有余地。可采用类似如下的表达：to the author's knowledge...，there is little information available in literature about...，until recently, there is some lack of knowledge about...，等等。

7．引言的最后部分可以阐明研究价值。理科方面的研究往往产生有价值的理论贡献，而工科方面的研究通常会有某些具体工程应用的前景。若是理论上的贡献，则要写出自己的研究结果能协助某些领域中的研究者说明某种现象、解决某个理论问题或为他们提供未来的研究方向。若有实际应用价值，则需说明自己的研究结果能协助某个领域的专业人员解决某些应用上的问题或达到某些目标。一般而言，专业研究人员习惯以谦虚或试探性的态度来指出自己研究的价值。例如，作者很少直接说明自己的研究结果能完全解决某个问题，即使作者对自己的研究结果非常有信心，也只会表示这些结果能"帮助"我们解决某个问题，或能提供一种"可能"的答案。为了表达这种谦虚的态度，应常使用情态助动词。其中较常用的助动词是 may，其他常用的助动词还有 should 及 could。

8．引言的时态运用：①叙述有关现象或普遍事实时，句子的主要动词多使用现在时，如 little is known about X 或 little literature is available on X。②描述特定研究领域中最近的某种趋势，或者强调表示某些"最近"发生的事件对现在的影响时，常采用现在完成时，如 few studies have been done on X 或 little attention has been devoted to X。③在阐述作者本人研究目的的句子中应有类似 this paper, the experiment reported here 等词，以表示所涉及的内容是作者的工作，而不是其他学者过去的研究。例如，"In summary, previous methods are all extremely inefficient. Hence a new approach is developed to process the data more efficiently."就容易使读者产生误解，其中的第二句应修改为："In this paper, a new approach will be developed to process the data more efficiently."或者"This paper will present (presents) a new approach that process the data more efficiently."。

实例

以下是从一篇科技研究报告中摘录出来的典型的引言，该引言包括上文提到的步骤一到步骤四。

VO$_2$ Max Trainability and High Intensity Interval Training in Humans: A Meta-Analysis

步骤一：
背景资料

The benefits of an active lifestyle are well documented. Many of these benefits are also associated with higher levels of cardiorespiratory fitness (VO$_2$ max) which may exert protective effects that are independent of traditional risk factors. Additionally, for individuals with low physical fitness, even modest improvements in fitness can have substantial health benefits. However, some individuals may have a limited ability to increase their cardiorespiratory fitness (trainability) in response to endurance exercise training.

步骤二：
文献回顾

A key study advancing the idea that some humans have limited trainability comes from Bouchard et al. studying 483 sedentary white adults from 99 nuclear families who completed a standardized 20-week endurance training program. The subjects were trained three times per week on a treadmill. Initially, they were trained at a heart rate that correlated to 55% of their baseline VO$_2$ max for 30 minutes per session. Every two weeks the intensity and duration of the exercise was progressively increased until each subject was training for 50 minutes at a heart rate associated with 75% of their baseline VO$_2$ max. This level of intensity and duration was reached by the 14th week of training and maintained until the conclusion of the study. Using this approach, they found a mean increase in VO$_2$ max of ~ 0.4L·min^{-1} with a SD of >0.2L·min^{-1}. Additionally, 7% of subjects showed a gain of 0.1L·min^{-1} or less while 8% of subjects improved by 0.7L·min^{-1} or more.

步骤三：
指出问题

Based on this distribution of VO$_2$ max responses it appears that the "trainability" of at least some subjects is low or non-existent with little or no improvement in cardiorespiratory fitness in spite of 20 weeks of structured exercise training. These observations are in contrast to reports from smaller studies that have used either interval training (IT) or interval training in combination with continuous training (CT), which show more robust increases in VO$_2$ max with at least some evidence of marked responses in all subjects.

步骤四：
研究目的

In this context, we sought to explore the hypothesis that all subjects can show marked improvements in VO$_2$ max if training programs that include periods of high intensity (~90% of VO$_2$ max) exercise are used. A fundamental rationale underpinning our analysis is that the biology of VO$_2$ max trainability needs to be evaluated using regimens designed to maximize physiological adaptations. To test this hypothesis, we evaluated the changes in VO$_2$ max in response to interval training (IT) or combined IT and continuous training (CT) reported in 37 studies. We also sought to gain insight into the idea that shorter periods of IT might be either superior or more efficient in generating increases of VO$_2$ max in comparison to traditional continuous training.

练习

请指出下列引言中步骤一到步骤四所包含的句子。

Spectral Properties of Electromyographic and Mechanomyographic Signals During Dynamic Concentric and Eccentric Contractions of the Human Biceps Brachii Muscle

Electromyography (EMG) and mechanomyography (MMG) studies have described differences in MU control strategies during concentric and eccentric muscle actions. Greater EMG activation in concentric contractions compared to eccentric muscle actions has been reported in various muscles. Moreover, it has been suggested that increases in muscle force were influenced more by motor unit (MU) recruitment than by changes in firing rate during concentric muscle contractions, whereas eccentric torque is primarily modulated through changes in motor unit firing rate of biceps brachill and vastus medialis. Although it is controversial, some EMG studies examining MU recruitment during eccentric contractions have demonstrated a preferential recruitment of fast MUs over slow MUs. However, the effect of joint position during eccentric and concentric contractions was not clear. It has been shown that changes of joint angle associated with muscle length had a significant effect on the maximum muscle force production during isometric contractions. It is not clear how exactly surface EMG and MMG activities are altered by the joint angle during dynamic eccentric and concentric contractions. Measurement of muscle activation patterns during dynamic concentric and eccentric contractions in relation to the joint angle is important for understanding the basic mechanisms underlying motor control of limb movement, and very useful for constructing models of the neuromuscular control system.

Therefore, the purpose of the present study was to describe and examine the variations in activation strategies of MUs in biceps brachii (BB) through a range of joint motions during eccentric and concentric contractions by using surface EMG, MMG, and a combination of wavelet analysis and principal component analysis (PCA) of the EMG and MMG spectra. Wavelet analysis that is well defined in time and frequency resolution, with the non-linear scaling adjusted to the physiological response time of the muscle, was used to decompose EMG and MMG signals from dynamic concentric and eccentric contractions. Then a quantitative method, principal component analysis (PCA), was used to describe the contribution of high- and low-frequency contents within the signal. It has been shown that the high and low frequency contents within the EMG and MMG are associated with the recruitment of fast and slow MUs, respectively. Therefore, this type of analysis can be used to determine which types of muscle fiber are active during locomotion (Wakeling and Rozitis, 2004). The general hypotheses were (1) the elbow angle has an effect on MU recruitment patterns during concentric and eccentric contractions; (2) concentric and eccentric contractions may induce different motor control strategies which can be detected by differences in the time-frequency properties of the EMG and MMG signals.

7.4   Speaking: Conference Presentation—Examples

Introducing the Supporting Materials（介绍支持材料）

1. I think this part is the most difficult, so I'll explain it in greater detail.

2. I think this part of my paper is most important, so I plan to spend more time on it.

3. Please allow me to deal with this matter more extensively.

4. Being the most important part of my presentation, I will elaborate on it with more slides.

5. I will indicate the points briefly.

6. Limited by the time available, I can only give you a very brief account of this matter.

7. I don't think that I should describe the methods in detail, because they are included in the handout.

8. I will not go into detail on it.

9. This point has been talked about repeatedly in this symposium, so I am not going to spend too much time on it.

Explaining the Contents on the Slides（解释幻灯片的内容）

1. This slide demonstrates...

2. On this slide, you can see...

3. This curve in this slide shows...

4. This figure in this slide exhibits...

5. This table on this slide presents...

6. This diagram on this slide depicts...

7. This chart on this slide displaces...

8. The picture on this slide shows...

9. The photomicrograph on this slide shows...

10. The flowchart on this slide points out...

11. The circuit diagram on this slide represents...

12. This figure is taken from.., by Dr. Li.

13. This diagram is after that of Prof. Wang with some modification.

Unit 8   Biomedical Sensors

8.1   Text: Biomedical Sensors

Biomedical sensors have a vital importance in modern life. We live in an epoch of computerization for every field of life. As we all know, computers can only process the data. Data must be collected, stored if necessary, and transferred to a computer. Biomedical sensors are designed for collecting data. It might be necessary to collect data for inpatients in hospital environment, in home for homebound patients, or for outpatients. This is an equivalent of monitoring. Monitoring is a necessary activity in risky environments such as mining, diving, mountain climbing, and especially in all sorts of military and security actions. All of these broad application fields have common requirements. The biomedical sensor should be compact and should not force the wearer to leave the comfort zone. These common requirements suggest the smart (intelligent) textiles along with the notion of wearable.

The concept of a wearable device that is always attached to a person (i.e. that can constantly be carried, unlike a personal stereo), is comfortable and easy to keep and use, and is "as unobtrusive as clothing".[1] Wearable systems are quite non-obtrusive devices that allow physicians to overcome the limitations of ambulatory technology and provide a response to the need for monitoring individuals over weeks or even months.[2] They typically rely on wireless, miniature sensors enclosed in patches or bandages, or in items that can be worn, such as a ring or a shirt.

Wearable sensors have diagnostic, as well as monitoring applications. Their current capabilities include physiological and biochemical sensing, as well as motion sensing. It is hard to overstate the magnitude of the problems that these technologies might help solve. Physiological monitoring could help in both diagnosis and ongoing treatment of a vast number of individuals with neurological, cardiovascular and pulmonary diseases such as seizures, hypertension, dysthymia, and asthma. Home based motion sensing might assist in falls prevention and help maximize an individual's independence and community participation.

Wearable sensors are used to gather physiological and movement data thus enabling patient's status monitoring.[3] Sensors are deployed according to the clinical application of interest. Sensors to monitor vital signs (e.g. heart rate and respiratory rate) would be deployed, for instance, when monitoring patients with congestive heart failure or patients with chronic obstructive pulmonary disease undergoing clinical intervention. Sensors for movement data capturing would be deployed, for instance, in applications such as monitoring the effectiveness of home-based rehabilitation interventions in stroke survivors or the use of mobility assistive devices in older adults. Wireless communication is relied upon to transmit patient's data to a mobile phone or an access point and relay the information to a remote center via the Internet. Emergency situations (e.g. falls) are detected via data processing implemented throughout the system and an alarm message is sent to an emergency service center to provide immediate assistance to patients. Family members and caregivers are alerted in case of an emergency but could also be notified in other situations when the patient requires assistance with, for instance, taking his/her medications. Clinical personnel can remotely monitor patient's status and be alerted in case a medical decision has to be made.

Despite the potential advantages of a remote monitoring system relying on wearable sensors like the one described above, there are significant challenges ahead before such a system can be utilized on a large scale.[4] These challenges include technological barriers such as limitations of currently available battery technology as well as cultural barriers such as the association of a stigma with the use of medical devices for home-based clinical monitoring.

Glossary

inpatient ['ɪnˌpeɪʃənt]	*n.* 住院病人
outpatient ['aʊtˌpeɪʃənt]	*n.* 门诊病人
unobtrusive [ˌʌnəb'truːsɪv]	*adj.* 不引人注目的
ambulatory ['æmbjələtɔrɪ]	*adj.* 流动的
bandage ['bændɪdʒ]	*n.* 绷带
diagnostic [ˌdaɪəg'nɒstɪk]	*adj.* 诊断的
pulmonary ['pʊlmənəri]	*adj.* 肺的，肺部的
dysthymia [dɪs'θaɪmɪə]	*n.* 精神抑郁（症）
asthma ['æsmə]	*n.* 气喘，哮喘
congestive [kən'dʒɛstɪv]	*adj.* 充血的
stigma ['stɪgmə]	*n.* 耻辱、羞辱

Technical Terms

biomedical sensor	生物医学传感器
comfort zone	舒适地带
personal stereo	随身听
wearable system	可穿戴系统
clinical intervention	临床干预

Notes

1. The concept of a wearable device that is always attached to a person (i.e. that can constantly be carried, unlike a personal stereo), is comfortable and easy to keep and use, and is "as unobtrusive as clothing".

与随身听不同，附着在人身上的可穿戴设备应具有舒适、易于保存和使用的特点，并且穿戴起来要像穿衣服那样自然。

分析：as...as...意思是"和……一样"，为同级比较，第一个 as 为副词，第二个 as 为连词。

2. Wearable systems are quite non-obtrusive devices that allow physicians to overcome the limitations of ambulatory technology and provide a response to the need for monitoring individuals over weeks or even months.

可穿戴系统是一种并不引人注目的设备，该系统可以使医生克服移动技术的局限性，并能对需要在数周甚至数月内监测个人数据这一需求做出回应。

分析：that 作关系代词引导定语从句，修饰 devices。

3. Wearable sensors are used to gather physiological and movement data thus enabling patient's status monitoring.

可穿戴传感器用于收集生理和运动数据，使得对患者状态的监测得以实现。

分析：thus 为副词，意为"因此，从而"，相当于 as a result、as a consequence of this、therefore 等。

4. Despite the potential advantages of a remote monitoring system relying on wearable sensors like the one described above, there are significant challenges ahead before such a system can be utilized on a large scale.

尽管依赖于上述可穿戴传感器的远程监控系统具有潜在的优势，但其在大规模使用之前还存在着重大的挑战。

分析：despite 用作介词时，与 in spite of 同义，都表示"尽管""虽然""不顾"之意。放在句首时，要接名词或名词词组充当成分。

Translation Skills：词义的选择

一词多类、一词多义是英汉两种语言中常见的语言现象。越是常用的词，越是拥有繁多的词义或属于不同的词类。正确的词义只有在具体的上下文中才能确定。一词多类就是指一个词属于几个词类，具有几个不同的意义，如英语中的 increase 既可以作动词，又可以作名词。一词多义就是说同一个词在同一个词类中有几个不同的词义，如英语中的 light 一词，用作名词时既指"光亮、光线"，又可以指"日光、白昼""发光体、光源""引火物、点火物""目光、眼神""眼光、观点"等。在进行英汉翻译时，词义选择是一项自始至终的思维活动，应根据词类、专业、搭配习惯、文体以及感情色彩、上下文等因素进行选择。

1. 根据多义词在句中的词类属性来确定词义

以 like 为例。

He likes running. （动词）
他喜欢跑步。

It doesn't look like it's going to rain. （介词）
看起来不像要下雨的样子。

Like charges repel; unlike charges attract. （形容词）
相同的电荷相斥，不同的电荷相吸。

Like knows like. （名词）
英雄识英雄。

2．根据专业选择词义

在英汉两种语言中，同一个词在不同的学科领域往往具有不同的词义。因此在选择词义时应考虑到原文中的内容所涉及的概念属于哪一类学科或专业。

① power

例句

Computers are a rising <u>power</u>.
计算机是一股正在蓬勃发展的<u>力量</u>。

The internal resistance of an ideal voltage <u>power</u> is close to zero.
理想电压<u>源</u>的内阻接近于零。

The <u>second power</u> of 3 is 9.
3 的<u>平方</u>（2 次方）是 9。

<u>Power</u> is the work done per unit of time.
<u>功率</u>是指单位时间所做的功。

<u>Electric power</u> is a kind of important energy.
<u>电力</u>是一种十分重要的能源。

In short, the <u>power</u> of the people is infinite.
总之，人民的<u>力量</u>是无限的。

② as

例句

The volume varies <u>as</u> the temperature increases.
体温<u>随着</u>温度增加而变化。（as 引导时间状语从句）

Small <u>as</u> atoms are, electrons are still smaller.
原子<u>虽然</u>很小，但电子更小。（as 引导让步状语从句）

<u>As</u> heat makes things move, it is a form of energy.
<u>由于</u>热能使物体运动，因此热是一种能量。（as 引导原因状语从句）

3．根据上下文选择词义

① aggressive

例句

<u>Aggressive</u> nations threaten world peace.
<u>有侵略性的</u>国家威胁世界和平。

A good salesman must be <u>aggressive</u> if he wants to succeed.
要做个好推销员一定要<u>有闯劲儿</u>，这样他才能成功。

② last

例句

He is the <u>last</u> man to come.

他是<u>最后来</u>的。

He is the <u>last</u> man to do it.

他<u>绝对不会</u>干那件事。

He is the <u>last</u> person for such a job.

他<u>最不配</u>干这个工作。

4．根据感情色彩选择词义

英语中有些词义是中立的，本身不表示褒义或贬义，但在一定的上下文中可能有褒贬的意味，在翻译时就应该用具有感情色彩的相应的词来表达。

例句

You're <u>flattering</u> me by saying that.

你那么说，就<u>过奖</u>了。（中性）

Hans was too obviously <u>flattering</u> the gentleman by saying he was the most courageous man he had ever seen.

汉斯说，这位先生是他所见到过的最有胆识的人，这种<u>阿谀奉承</u>未免过于露骨。（贬义）

He had lied to me and made me the tool of his wicked <u>deeds</u>.

他欺骗了我，使我成了他进行罪恶<u>勾当</u>的工具。（贬义）

His heroic <u>deeds</u> were celebrated in every corner of China.

全国各地的人们都在颂扬他的英雄<u>事迹</u>。（褒义）

5．根据搭配习惯选择词义

① heavy

■ heavy current

例句

This electric motor is working in full under the action of <u>heavy current</u>.

在<u>强电流</u>的作用下，这台电机正以满荷运行。

■ heavy industry

例句

The salary-employment mechanism under traditional system gives priority to the development of <u>heavy industry</u>.

传统体制下的工资与就业制度是为优先发展<u>重工业</u>这一战略而服务的。

■ heavy traffic

例句

In order to avoid the <u>heavy traffic</u> on the roads, some people prefer to travel by night and rest during the day.

为了避免路上<u>交通拥堵</u>，有些人宁可夜间驱车远行，白天用来休息。

② apply

■ apply for

例句

He decided to <u>apply for</u> the job.
他决定<u>申请</u>这个职位。

■ apply to

例句

Our teacher <u>applies</u> this teaching method <u>to</u> his class.
我们老师把这种教学方法<u>应用到</u>他的班级。

8.2   Listening: Biosensors

Section 1

A biosensor is an analytical device, used for the detection of an analyte, which combines a biological component with a physicochemical detector. The sensitive biological element, e.g. tissue, microorganisms, organelles, cell receptors, enzymes, antibodies, nucleic acids, etc., is a biologically derived material or biomimetic component that interacts, binds, or recognizes with the analyte under study. The biologically sensitive elements can also be created by biological engineering. The transducer or the detector element, which transforms one signal into another one, works in a physicochemical way: optical, piezoelectric, electrochemical, electrochemiluminescence etc. The biosensor reader device functions with the associated electronics or signal processors that are primarily responsible for the display of the results in a user-friendly way. This sometimes accounts for the most expensive part of the sensor device, however it is possible to generate a user-friendly display that includes transducer and sensitive element (holographic sensor). The readers are usually custom-designed and manufactured to suit the different working principles of biosensors.

Section 2

There are many potential applications of biosensors. The main requirements for a biosensor approach to be valuable in terms of research and commercial applications are the identification of a target molecule, availability of a suitable biological recognition element, and the potential for disposable portable detection systems to be preferred to sensitive laboratory-based techniques in some situations. Some examples are glucose monitoring in diabetes patients, other medical health related targets, environmental applications (e.g. the detection of pesticides and river water contaminants such as heavy metal ions), remote sensing of airborne bacteria (e.g. in counter-bioterrorist activities), remote sensing of water quality in coastal waters by describing online different aspects of clam ethology (e.g. biological rhythms, growth rates, spawning or death records) in groups of abandoned bivalves around the world, detection of pathogens, determining levels of toxic substances before and after bioremediation, detection and determining of organophosphate, routine analytical measurement of folic acid, biotin, vitamin B12 and pantothenic acid as an alternative to microbiological assay, determination of drug residues in food, such as antibiotics and growth promoters, particularly meat and honey, drug discovery and evaluation of biological activity of new compounds, protein engineering in biosensors, and detection of toxic metabolites such as mycotoxins.

🎧 Section 3

A common example of a commercial biosensor is the blood glucose biosensor, which uses the enzyme glucose oxidase to break blood glucose down. In doing so it first oxidizes glucose and uses two electrons to reduce the FAD (a component of the enzyme) to FADH2. This in turn is oxidized by the electrode in a number of steps. The resulting current is a measure of the concentration of glucose. In this case, the electrode is the transducer and the enzyme is the biologically active component.

A canary in a cage, as used by miners to warn of gas, could be considered a biosensor. Many of today's biosensor applications are similar, in that they use organisms which respond to toxic substances at a much lower concentrations than humans can detect to warn of their presence. Such devices can be used in environmental monitoring, trace gas detection and in water treatment facilities.

◆ *Source: https://en.wikipedia.org/wiki/Biosensor.*

Listening Exercises

Listen to each section twice, and as you are listening, (a) number the words or expressions in the list on the work sheet by order of their first appearance in the passage you are listening to; (b) check if your numbering is correct—if incorrect, listen to the section again; (c) orally answer the questions about the content of each section.

Unit 8, Section 1

analyte	biomimetic	principles
antibodies	electrochemiluminescence	results
associated	physiochemical	transducer

1. How does an analyte work?

2. What is the role of the transducer or detector element?

3. What is generally the most expensive part of the sensor device?

Unit 8, Section 2

contaminants	mycotoxins	requirements
discovery	pathogens	spawning
disposable	remote sensing	targets

1. What are the main requirements for a biosensor to be effective?

2. Can you think of a medical situation where one would prefer a disposable portable device rather than laboratory-based techniques?

3. Name two types of food that should be examined for drug residues.

Unit 8, section 3

blood glucose	environmental	oxidizes
canary	enzyme	transducer
current	organisms	warn

1. What is the biologically active component in a blood glucose biosensor?

2. Name a living vertebrate that could be considered a biosensor.

3. How does that biosensor alert the users when a dangerous substance is present?

8.3　Writing: Materials and Methods

在论文中，这一部分用于说明实验的对象、条件、使用的材料、实验步骤或计算的过程、公式的推导、模型的建立等。对过程的描述要完整具体，符合逻辑，以便能够重复实验。

具体要求及内容

1. 对材料和设备的描述应清楚、准确。材料描述部分应该清楚地指出研究对象（样品或产品、动物、植物、病人）的数量、来源和准备方法。对于实验材料的名称，应采用国际同行所熟悉的通用名，尽量避免使用只有作者所在国家通用的专门名称。设备描述部分应包括仪器设备的名称及生产制造公司，对于特殊实验设备需要详细介绍。

2. 对实验过程的介绍。

3. 对统计分析方法的描述（一般情况下作者会把这些资料放在方法部分中，但少数的作者习惯把它放在结果部分）。

4. 对方法的描述要详略得当、重点突出。应遵循的原则是要给出足够的细节信息以便让读者能够重复实验，避免混入有关结果或发现方面的内容。如果方法新颖且不曾发表过，应提供所有必需的细节；如果所采用的方法已经公开报道过，则引用相关的文献即可（如果报道该方法的期刊的影响力很有限，可稍加详细地描述）。

5. 力求语法正确、描述准确。由于材料和方法部分通常需要描述很多的内容，因此需采用简洁的语言，使英语用词精确。需要注意的方面通常有如下几点。

① 不要遗漏动作的执行者，如 to determine its respiratory quotient, the organism was...，显然"the organism"不能"determine"；又如 having completed the study, the bacteria were of no further interest，显然，"the bacteria"不会"completed the study"。

② 在追求简洁表达的同时要注意内容方面的逻辑性，如 blood samples were taken from 48 informed and consenting patients...the subjects ranged in age from 6 months to 22 years，其中的语法没有错误，但六个月（6 months）的婴儿如何能表达自己同意参加实验的意愿呢？该例句显然欠缺逻辑性。

③ 如果有多种可供选择的方法，在引用文献时应提及一下具体的方法，如 cells were broken as previously described 不够清楚明确，应将其改为 cells were broken by ultrasonic treatment as previously described。

6．时态与语态的运用

① 若描述的内容为不受时间影响的事实，应采用一般现在时，如 a twin-lens reflex camera is actually a combination of two separate camera boxes。

② 若描述的内容为特定、过去的行为或事件，则采用一般过去时，如 the work was carried out on the Imperial College gas atomizer, which has been described in detail elsewhere。

③ 方法章节的焦点在于描述实验中进行的每个步骤以及采用的材料。由于涉及的步骤与材料是讨论的焦点，而且读者已经知道进行这些行为和采用这些材料的人就是作者，因而一般都习惯使用被动语态。例如，

优：The samples were immersed in an ultrasonic bath for 3 minutes in acetone followed by 10 minutes in distilled water.

劣：We immersed the samples in an ultrasonic bath for 3 minutes in acetone followed by 10 minutes in distilled water.

④ 在表达作者的观点或看法时，则应采用主动语态。例如，

优：For the second trial, the apparatus was covered by a sheet of plastic. We believed this modification would reduce the amount of scattering.

劣：For the second trial, the apparatus was covered by a sheet of plastic. It was believed that this modification would reduce the amount of scattering.

8.4　Speaking: Conference Presentation—Examples

Ending（结束）

1. Let's look at what I have talked about.

2. Well, that brings me to the end of my presentation. This last slide is a brief summary of what I have talked about.

3. Before I stop/finish, let me just say...

4. To close my speech, I'll show you the last slide.

5. Now I'd like to summarize my talk.

6. To summarize, I have talked about three aspects of the cancer problem: ...

7. Finally, as a summary statement, I would like to sum up the major points I have made.

Summary（总结）

1. Let me just run over the key points again.

2. I'll briefly summarize the main issues.

3. In conclusion,...

4. In closing,...

5. In a word,…

6. To sum up,…

7. In brief,…

8. Briefly,…

9. All in all,…

Conclusion （结论）

1. As you can see, there are some very good reasons ...

2. To sum up, my conclusion is that the present program is the best one.

3. In conclusion, ...

4. Let me conclude my talk with the following comments.

5. Allow me to conclude by listing out all the factors influencing the efficacy.

6. In conclusion, I would like to point out the following aspects.

7. I'd like to leave you with the following conclusion.

Closing （结束语）

1. That's all, thank you.

2. That's the end of my presentation.

3. So much for my speech, thank you.

4. Thank you for your attention.

5. Thank you for your listening.

Unit 9　Biosignal Processing

9.1　Text: Biosignal Processing

Any signal transduced from a biological or medical source could be called a biosignal. The signal source could be at the molecular level, cell level, or a systemic or organ level. A wide variety of such signals are commonly encountered in the clinic, research laboratory, and sometimes even at home. Examples include the electrocardiogram (ECG), or electrical activity from the heart; speech signals; the electroencephalogram (EEG), or electrical activity from the brain; evoked potentials (EPs, i.e., auditory, visual, somatosensory, etc.), or electrical responses of the brain to specific peripheral stimulation; the electroneurogram, or field potentials from local regions in the brain; action potential signals from individual neurons or heart cells; the electromyogram (EMG), or electrical activity from the muscle; the electroretinogram from the eye; and so on.

Clinically, biomedical signals are primarily acquired for monitoring (detecting or estimating) specific pathological/physiological states for purposes of diagnosis and evaluating therapy. In some cases of basic research, they are also used for decoding and eventual modeling of specific biological systems. Furthermore, current technology allows the acquisition of multiple channels of these signals. This brings up additional signal-processing challenges to quantify physiologically meaningful interactions among these channels.

Goals of signal processing in all these cases usually are noise removal, accurate quantification of signal model and its components through analysis (system identification for modeling and control purposes), feature extraction for deciding function or dysfunction, and prediction of future pathological or functional events as in prosthetic devices for heart and brain. Typical biological applications may involve the use of signal-processing algorithms for more than one of these reasons. The monitored biological signal in most cases is considered an additive combination of signal and noise. Noise can be from instrumentation (sensors, amplifiers, filters, etc.), from electromagnetic interference (EMI), or in general, any signal that is asynchronous and uncorrelated with the underlying physiology of interest.[1] Therefore different situations warrant different assumptions for noise characteristics, which will eventually lead to an appropriate choice of signal-processing method.

Biomedical signals can be classified according to various characteristics of the signal, including the waveform shape, statistical structure, and temporal properties. Two broad classes of signals that are commonly encountered include continuous and discrete signals. Continuous signals are defined over a continuum of time or space and are described by continuous variable functions. Signals that are produced by biological phenomena are almost always continuous signals. Some examples include voltage measurements from the heart, arterial blood pressure measurements, and measurements of electrical activity from the brain. Unlike continuous signals, which are defined along a continuum of points in space or time, discrete signals are defined only at a subset of regularly spaced points in time and/or space. Although most biological signals are not discrete per se, discrete signals play an important role due to today's advancements in digital technology. Sophisticated medical instruments are commonly used to convert continuous signals from the human body to discrete digital sequences that can be analyzed and interpreted with a computer.[2]

Biological signals can also be classified as being either deterministic or random. Deterministic signals can be described by mathematical functions or rules. Periodic and transient signals make up a subset of all deterministic signals. Real biological signals almost always have some unpredictable noise or change in parameters and, therefore, are not entirely deterministic. Random signals, also called stochastic signals, contain uncertainty in the parameters that describe them. Because of this uncertainty, mathematical functions cannot be used to precisely describe random signals. Instead, random signals are most often analyzed using statistical techniques that require the treatment of the random parameters of the signal with probability distributions or simple statistical measures such as the mean and standard deviation. The electromyogram (EMG), an electrical recording of electrical activity in skeletal muscle that is used for the diagnosis of neuromuscular disorders, is a random signal. Stationary random signals are signals for which the statistics or frequency spectra remain constant over time. Conversely, nonstationary random signals have statistical properties or frequency spectra that vary with time. In many instances, the identification of stationary segments of random signals is important for proper signal processing, pattern analysis, and clinical diagnosis.

◆ *Source: Standard handbook of biomedical engineering and design; Introduction to biomedical engineering.*

Glossary

molecular [mə'lekjʊlə]	*adj.* 分子的
electrocardiograph [ɪˌlektrəʊ'kɑːdɪəgrɑːf]	*n.* 心电图仪
electroencephalogram [ɪˌlektrəʊɪn'sefələgræm]	*n.* 脑电图
somatosensory [soˌmætə'sensəri]	*n.* 躯体感觉
peripheral [pə'rɪfərəl]	*adj.* 外围的
electromyogram [ɪˌlektroˌmaɪəˌgræm]	*n.* 肌电图
electroretinogram [ɪˌlektro'retənəgræm]	*n.* 网膜电图
pathological [ˌpæθə'lɒdʒɪkəl]	*adj.* 病理学的
dysfunction [dɪs'fʌŋkʃən]	*n.* 功能障碍
asynchronous [eɪ'sɪŋkrənəs]	*adj.* 异步的
per se [ˌpɜː'seɪ]	*adv.* 本身，本质上
nonstationary [ˌnɒn'steɪʃənəri]	*adj.* 非平稳的

Technical Terms

evoked potentials	诱发电位
electromagnetic interference	电磁干扰
temporal property	时间特性
stochastic signals	随机信号
probability distributions	概率分布
statistical property	统计特征
frequency spectra	频谱

Notes

1. Noise can be from instrumentation (sensors, amplifiers, filters, etc.), from electromagnetic interference (EMI), or in general, any signal that is asynchronous and uncorrelated with the underlying physiology of interest.

噪声可能来自仪表（传感器、放大器、滤波器等），可能来自电磁干扰（EMI），或一般来说，来自任何异步的、与潜在的生理机能无关的信号。

分析：that 引导定语从句，修饰 signal。此句中包含并列结构，from instrumentation，from electromagnetic interference 及 or in general…并列表达噪声的三个来源。

2. Sophisticated medical instruments are commonly used to convert continuous signals from the human body to discrete digital sequences that can be analyzed and interpreted with a computer.

复杂的医疗仪器通常用于将人体的连续信号转换为离散的数字序列，这些数字序列可以通过计算机进行分析和解释。

分析：that 引导限定性定语从句，修饰 digital sequences。

Translation Skills：句型的转换

在翻译的过程中，可以根据原文的具体情况，按照汉语的表达习惯，对原文句子结构进行调整和转换。常见的转换方式有以下几种。

1. 否定变肯定译法

该方法会将原文中的否定表达形式译成肯定形式。

例句

<u>No</u> one had known about the good properties of the device <u>until</u> that experiment was made.
只有经过那个实验后，人们才了解了这台装置的优良性能。

The fuel or lubricant <u>cannot</u> be sold <u>until</u> they are separated and purified of any contaminants and impurities.
只有经过分离过滤掉污染物和杂质，燃油或润滑油才可以出售。

2. 肯定变否定译法

该方法是将原文中的肯定表达形式译成否定形式。

🌱例句

All problems in this project are <u>too difficult to be solved</u>.

这个工程的一切问题都<u>难得无法解决</u>。

There are many other energy sources <u>in store</u>.

还有多种其他能源<u>尚未开发</u>。

3. 主动变被动译法

在具体论文中，如果将原文主动句从正面译出比较困难，或者将其译成汉语被动句后更能准确地表达原义、使得汉语行文更为流畅时，可把原文主动句译成汉语的被动句。

🌱例句

The properties of materials <u>have dictated</u> nearly every design and every useful application that the engineer could devise.

工程师所能设想的每一种设计和每一种用途几乎都<u>受到</u>材料性能的<u>限制</u>。

Since prehistoric times the sketch <u>has served as</u> one of man's most effective communication techniques.

从史前时期以来，草图一直<u>被</u>人类<u>当作</u>最有效的交际手段之一。

9.2　Listening: Biosignal and Digital Image Processing

🎧 Section 1

A biosignal is any signal in living beings that can be continually measured and monitored. The term biosignal is often used to refer to bioelectrical signals, but it may refer to both electrical and non-electrical signals. The usual understanding is to refer only to time-varying signals, although spatial parameter variations (e.g. the nucleotide sequence determining the genetic code) are sometimes subsumed as well.

Electrical biosignals, or bioelectrical time signals, usually refers to the change in electric current produced by the sum of an electrical potential difference across a specialized tissue, organ or cell system like the nervous system. Thus, among the best-known bioelectrical signals are:

- Electroencephalogram (EEG);
- Electrocardiogram (ECG);
- Electromyogram (EMG);
- Mechanomyogram (MMG);
- Electrooculogram (EOG);
- Galvanic skin response (GSR);
- Magnetoencephalogram (MEG).

EEG, ECG, EOG and EMG are measured with a differential amplifier which registers the difference between two electrodes attached to the skin. However, the galvanic skin response measures electrical resistance and the MEG measures the magnetic field induced by electrical currents (electroencephalogram) of the brain.

Section 2

With the development of methods for remote measurement of electric fields using new sensor technology, electric biosignals such as EEG and ECG can be measured without electric contact with the skin. This can be applied for example for remote monitoring of brain waves and heart beat of patients who must not be touched, in particular patients with serious burns.

Electrical currents and changes in electrical resistances across tissues can also be measured from plants.

Biosignals may also refer to any non-electrical signal that is capable of being monitored from biological beings, such as mechanical signals (e.g. the mechanomyogram or MMG), acoustic signals (e.g. phonetic and non-phonetic utterances, breathing), chemical signals (e.g. pH, oxygenation) and optical signals (e.g. movements).

Section 3

Medical image computing (MIC) is an interdisciplinary field at the intersection of computer science, data science, electrical engineering, physics, mathematics and medicine. This field develops computational and mathematical methods for solving problems pertaining to medical images and their use for biomedical research and clinical care.

The main goal of MIC is to extract clinically relevant information or knowledge from medical images. While closely related to the field of medical imaging, MIC focuses on the computational analysis of the images, not their acquisition. The methods can be grouped into several broad categories: image segmentation, image registration, image-based physiological modeling, and others.

Segmentation is the process of partitioning an image into different meaningful segments. In medical imaging, these segments often correspond to different tissue classes, organs, pathologies, or other biologically relevant structures. Medical image segmentation is made difficult by low contrast, noise, and other imaging ambiguities. Although there are many computer vision techniques for image segmentation, some have been adapted specifically for medical image computing.

Image registration is a process that searches for the correct alignment of images. In the simplest case, two images are aligned. Typically, one image is treated as the target image and the other is treated as a source image; the source image is transformed to match the target image. The optimization procedure updates the transformation of the source image based on a similarity value that evaluates the current quality of the alignment. This iterative procedure is repeated until a (local) optimum is found.

◆ *Source: https://en.wikipedia.org/wiki/Biosignal.*

Listening Exercises

Listen to each section twice, and as you are listening, (a) number the words or expressions in the list on the work sheet by order of their first appearance in the passage you are listening to; (b) check if your numbering is correct—if incorrect, listen to the section again; (c) orally answer the questions about the content of each section.

Unit 9, Section 1

beings	galvanic	subsumed
bioelectrical	magnetoencephalogram	time signals
electroencephalogram	mechanomyogram	time-varying

1. What are the two biosignals distinguished in this article?
2. What is the main parameter variation in a biosignal?
3. Name three well-known bioelectrical time signals.

Unit 9, Section 2

acoustic	in particular	oxygenation
breathing	measurement	remote
electric	non-electrical	resistances

1. Name a case where it is important to measure brain waves or heart beat remotely.
2. Give two examples of non-electrical biosignals.

Unit 9, Section 3

alignment	correspond	pertaining
ambiguities	grouped	relevant
computational	optimum	target

1. What is developed by a specialist in medical image processing?
2. Does medical image processing focus on data acquisition?
3. What makes medical image segmentation difficult?

9.3   Writing: Results

本部分描述研究结果的写作。研究结果通常自成体系，也就是说，读者不必参考论文其他部分，也能了解作者的研究成果。对结果的叙述也要按照其逻辑顺序进行，使之既符合实验过程的逻辑顺序，又符合实验结果的推导过程。结果部分还可以包括对实验结果的分类整理和对比分析等。

写作要求

1．对实验或观察结果的表达要高度概括和提炼，不能简单地将实验数据或观察到的事实堆积到论文中。尤其要突出有科学意义和具有代表性的数据，而不是一再地重复一般性数据。

2．对实验结果的叙述要客观真实，即使得到的结果与实验不符，也不可略而不述，而且还应在讨论中加以说明和解释。

3．数据表达可采用文字与图表相结合的形式。如果只有一个或很少的测定结果，在正文中用文字描述即可；如果数据较多，可采用图表的形式对其进行完整、详细地列举，文字部分则用来指出图表中资料的重要特性或趋势。切忌在文字中简单地重复图表中的数据，而忽略叙述其趋势、意义以及相关推论。

4．适当解释原始数据，以帮助读者理解。尽管对于研究结果的详细讨论主要出现在讨论部分，但在结果部分应该提及必要的解释，以便让读者清楚地了解作者此次研究结果的意义或重要性。

5．文字表达应准确、简洁、清楚。避免使用繁复的词或句子来介绍或解释图表。为简洁、清楚起见，不要把图表的序号作为段落的主题句，应在句子中指出图表所揭示的结论，并把图表的序号放入括号中。例如，Figure 1 shows the relationship between A and B 不如 A was significantly higher than B at all time points hecked (Figure 1)。又如，it is clearly shown in Table 1 that nocillin inhibited the growth of N. gonorrhoeae 不如 nocillin inhibited the growth of N. gonorrhoeae (Table 1)。

6．时态的运用应遵循以下原则。

■ 指出结果在哪些图表中列出，常用一般现在时，如 Figure 2 shows the variation in the temperature of the samples over time。

■ 叙述或总结研究结果的内容为关于过去的事实，所以通常采用一般过去时，如 after flights of less than two hours, 11% of the army pilots and 33% of the civilian pilots reported back pain。

■ 在对研究结果进行说明或由其得出一般性推论时，多用一般现在时，如 the higher incidence of back pain in civilian pilots may be due to their greater accumulated flying time。

■ 在不同结果之间或实验数据与理论模型之间进行比较时，多采用一般现在时（这种比较关系多为不受时间影响的逻辑上的事实），如 these results agree well with the findings of Smith, et al。

举例

Incidence of Back Pain in Helicopter Pilots Results

Table 1 presents the data on the prevalence of back pain directly associated with flight. Particularly high back pain prevalence were reported after flights of more than 2 hours or after a period of intensive flying. Moreover, civilian pilots, with their greater accumulated flight time, reported a greater prevalence of back pain after flights of all durations. It appears that both the flight duration and total accumulated flight time affect the incidence of back pain.

Table 1.　Prevalence of back pain directly associated with flight time

	Army pilots (n=87)		Civilian pilots (n=39)	
	%	(abs)	%	(abs)
After or during each fight	11	(9)	14	(5)
A fight <2h	11	(9)	33	(11)
A fight >2h	35	(28)	72	(26)
A fight with a high level of concentration	30	(24)	53	(18)
Period >20h a week	48	(38)	74	(26)

　　在上面的例子中，段落中的第一个句子介绍作者将讨论的资料，并告诉读者这些数据在哪个图表中可以看到。第二句和第三句则叙述最重要的结果。第四句为关于这些结果的评论——在此例子中，评论的内容为根据 Table 1 中的资料得出的推论。

注意事项

　　在描述上面表格中的数据时，作者并没有列出所有的数据，而只是指出了这些资料中体现的两个重要的事实。在撰写研究论文时，应避免在论文和图表中提出一模一样的内容，而且千万不要在论文中重复图表中的所有数据。详细的结果应采用图表来表示，同时利用论文来指出图表中数据的重要特性或趋势。在介绍研究结果时，作者应为读者诠释自己的结果，不要在图表中把一大堆数据列出来而让读者自己去解读这些数据。作者应该直接告诉读者这些数据出现什么样的趋势、具有什么意义。在结果部分中应该对研究结果提供一些基本的解释，以便让读者清楚、容易地了解在此次研究中究竟得到了什么样的结果。

　　最后，研究报告的图表应尽可能地清晰明了，以便读者在没有看到论文的情况下也能大致了解图表的内容。例如，图表应有清楚的标题与标记。

9.4　Speaking: Tips for Chinese Presenters at International Conferences

　　非英语母语的人在做英文会议报告时，会遇到一些特殊的问题。本节将介绍一些方法来帮助大家顺利地完成会议报告。

　　1．多用简单的英文单词组成简短的句子。在报告中尽量不要使用如 following the addition of oxygen, the hardness of the samples was observed to increase significantly 这样的长句，而应该说 adding oxygen made the samples much harder。

　　2．在做报告时，声音要洪亮，发音要清晰。

　　3．在做报告时语速要慢。要常常提醒自己：慢，慢，再慢！

　　4．英文单词中的元音发音要饱满。中国人说英语时，在发音方面最明显的缺点之一，是常常把所有的英文元音都"切断"，尤其是短音的发音更是如此。在说英文时，需要放松喉咙，并把元音的声音拉长。喉咙放松后，英文发音才会自然。

5．英文单词的每一个音节都需要发音清晰，尤其是当字尾为辅音时，更需注意这一点。中国人说英文时另一个常犯的错误，是英文单词的最后一个音节或字母根本没有发音。如果希望听众了解我们的意思，则必须把完整的音节都发出来，不能任意省略其中某个音节。

6．在说话时要使用完整的句子——具有主语和动词等成分的独立句子。所说的句子可以很简短，但都应该是完整的。

7．多学习自己专业领域中常用英文单词的正确发音，尤其是当不知道单词的哪个音节为重音时，应该查辞典确定。若可能的话，可以请英文为母语的朋友、同事或英语老师试听自己的演讲，并纠正演讲中任何发音不正确的单词。

要加强或改善自己的英文发音，最好是"立即"开始。也就是说，我们不要等到做会议报告前的最后一个星期，才开始注意自己英文发音的问题。在遇到发音比较困难或复杂的英文单词或在书上看到生词时，应该随时翻阅辞典，以查出正确的发音方法与重音位置。

8．应该把自己会议报告中的所有关键词都放入幻灯片中。如果某个重要单词的发音不标准，听众还能在幻灯片上看到这个单词。

9．在做英文会议报告时，不要担心自己的英语是否有文法错误，重要的是自己的表达技巧、报告内容要达到专业水平，而且发音也要清晰。只要将报告的重点表达清楚，听众应该可以忽略一些语法上的小错误。他们所关心的是我们是否能以清晰的方式对大家感兴趣的题目提供一些有用的信息。

要记住，熟能生巧。经过大量的练习和精心的准备，大家用英语做报告的能力一定会得到提高。在应用英语和全世界同行交流学科前沿的过程中，可以帮助我们结交来自不同国家的朋友和潜在的合作者。

Unit 10　Biomedical Instrumentation

10.1　Text: Biomedical Instrumentation

The major difference between medical instrumentation and conventional instrumentation systems is that the source of signals is living tissue or energy applied to living tissue.[1] The principal measurement and frequency ranges for each medical and physiological parameter are major factors that affect the design of all the instrument components. Most of the medical parameter measurement ranges are quite low compared with nonmedical parameters. Note, for example, that most voltages are in the microvolt range and that pressures are low (about 100 mm Hg=1.93 psi =13.3 kPa). Also note that all the signals listed are in the audio-frequency range or below and that many signals contain direct current (DC) and very low frequencies.[2] These general properties of medical parameters limit the practical choices available to designers for all aspects of instrument design.

Crucial variables in living systems are inaccessible because the proper measurand-sensor interface cannot be obtained without damaging the system. Unlike many complex physical systems, a biological system is of such a nature that it is not possible to turn it off and remove parts of it during the measurement procedure.[3] Even if interference from other physiological systems can be avoided, the physical size of many sensors prohibits the formation of a proper interface. Either such inaccessible variables must be measured indirectly, or corrections must be applied to data that are affected by the measurement process. The cardiac output is an important measurement that is obviously quite inaccessible.

Variables measured from the human body or from animals are seldom deterministic. Many medical measurements vary widely among normal patients, even when conditions are similar. This inherent variability has been documented at the molecular and organ levels, and even for the whole body. Many internal anatomical variations accompany the obvious external differences among patients. Large tolerances on physiological measurements are partly the result of interactions among many physiological systems. Many feedback loops exist among physiological systems, and many of the interrelationships are poorly understood. It is seldom feasible to control or neutralize the effects of these other systems on the measured variable. The most common method of coping with this variability is to assume empirical statistical and probabilistic distribution functions.

Nearly all biomedical measurements depend either on some form of energy being applied to the living tissue or on some energy being applied as an incidental consequence of sensor operation. X-ray and ultrasonic imaging techniques and electromagnetic or Doppler ultrasonic blood flowmeters depend on externally applied energy interacting with living tissue. Safe levels of these various types of energy are difficult to establish, because many mechanisms of tissue damage are not well understood. A fetus is particularly vulnerable during the early stages of development. The heating of tissue is one effect that must be limited，because even reversible physiological changes can affect measurements. Damage to tissue at the molecular level has been demonstrated in some instances at surprisingly low energy levels.

Operation of instruments in the medical environment imposes important additional constraints. Equipment must be reliable, easy to operate, and capable of withstanding physical abuse and exposure to corrosive chemicals. Electronic equipment must be designed to minimize electric-shock hazards. The safety of patients and medical personnel must be considered in all phases of the design and testing of instruments.

◆ *Source: Medical Instrumentation Application and Design.*

Glossary

anatomical [ˌænə'tɒmɪkəl]　　　　*adj.* 解剖的
tolerance ['tɒlərəns]　　　　　　*n.* 容差
neutralize ['nju:trəlaɪz]　　　　　*v.* 抵消
ultrasonic [ˌʌltrə'sɒnɪk]　　　　*adj.* 超声波的
fetus ['fi:təs]　　　　　　　　　*n.* 胎儿

Technical Terms

microvolt range　　　　　　　　　　微伏范围
cardiac output　　　　　　　　　　　心输出量
inherent variability　　　　　　　　固有变异性
probabilistic distribution functions　概率分布函数
corrosive chemical　　　　　　　　　腐蚀剂
doppler ultrasonic blood flowmeter　多普勒超声血流量计

Notes

1. The major difference between medical instrumentation and conventional instrumentation systems is that the source of signals is living tissue or energy applied to living tissue.

医疗仪器和传统仪器的主要区别在于医疗仪器的信号源是活组织或应用于活组织的能量。

分析：that 引导表语从句。

2. Also note that all the signals listed are in the audio-frequency range or below and that many signals contain direct current (DC) and very low frequencies.

还要注意，所列的信号都在音频范围内或低于音频范围，因此许多信号包含直流（DC）和非常低的频率。

分析：that all…below 与 that many signals…low frequencies 均为 note 的宾语从句，由 that 引导。

3. Unlike many complex physical systems, a biological system is of such a nature that it is not possible to turn it off and remove parts of it during the measurement procedure.

与许多复杂的物理系统不同，生物系统具有这样的性质，因此在测量过程中不可能将其关闭或移除系统的某一部分。

分析：such…that 引导结果状语从句。

4. Either such inaccessible variables must be measured indirectly, or corrections must be applied to data that are affected by the measurement process.

我们要么间接测量这些不可直接获取的变量，要么必须对受测量过程影响的数据进行修正。

分析：that 引导定语从句，修饰 data。

Translation Skills：连接词的翻译

1. and

在英语中，and 是一个极为普遍的连接词，其基本意思是"和、又、而、及"。其实，and 在句中可以有多种特殊用法，表示多种意义，而且连接的不都是两个简单的并列成分。在实际翻译过程中，特别是在连接两个句子时，它的译法很多，表达意义不尽相同。如果不考虑 and 前后成分之间的逻辑关系，只用这几种译法生搬硬套，难免会造成理解上的失误，把整个句子的含义搞错。

（1）and 表示因果

例句

It follows that the unfavorable parameters are the impulsive force F and impulse frequency f, and anything that can be done to reduce either, or both, will be beneficial in reducing the maximum amplitude induced.

由此可见，不利参数是冲击力 F 和脉冲频率 f。<u>因此</u>，任何能减少其中之一或两者的措施都有利于降低感应的最大振幅。

Parameters extracted from such measures can provide indicators of health status <u>and</u> have tremendous diagnostic value.

从这些措施中提取的参数可以提供健康状况的指标，<u>所以</u>具有巨大的诊断价值。

For the alloy steels, the heat-treating processes are somewhat modified <u>and</u> often of more restricted scope than those possible with carbon steels.

对合金钢来说，热处理工艺要有所修改，这是<u>因为</u>对合金钢进行的热处理工艺范围往往比对碳钢可能进行的热处理工艺范围受到更多的限制。

（2）and 表示目的

例句

It was later shown that the results of this work were by no means the ultimate, and further work has been put in hand <u>and</u> to provide closer control and more consistent operation in the area.

后来有人指出，这项工作的结果绝不是最终的结果，并已着手进行进一步的工作，<u>以便</u>对该地区实施更密切的控制，采取更一致的行动。

Shall we go <u>and</u> have a cup of coffee?

我们出去喝杯咖啡好吗?

（3）and 表示承接

例句

The next usual step is to decide on the location of the filter <u>and</u> the choice may be influenced by some factors.

通常，下一个步骤是确定过滤器的位置，<u>而</u>位置的选择要受到某些因素的影响。

The necessary oxygen is taken in through the lungs <u>and</u> is carried to the cells by the red colour matter of the blood.

这里所需的氧气通过肺部吸入，<u>然后</u>通过血液中的血红素输送到细胞中。

The example shown in Figure 3 demonstrates how sensors can be embedded in a garment to collect, for instance, electrocardiographic and electromyographic data by weaving electrodes into the fabric and to gather movement data by printing conductive elastomer-based components on the fabric <u>and</u> then sensing changes in their resistance associated with stretching of the garment due to subject's movements.

图 3 所示的例子说明了如何将电极植入织物，从而将传感器嵌入衣服，以实现心电数据和肌电数据的收集等功能，以及如何通过在织物上印刷导电弹性体类物质，<u>然后</u>感测由于受试者的运动而导致的与衣服拉伸相关的阻力变化来收集运动数据。

（4）and 表示原因

例句

The window pane was obviously quite old, <u>and</u> it had waves through it.

这块窗户的玻璃显然有些年头了，<u>因为</u>表面已经有些不平整。

Laser is incredibly deadly, <u>and</u> in the blink of an eye, it can destroy the enemy's outer space communication satellites, shutting down much of their advanced intelligent system.

激光是非常致命的。眨眼之间，它可以摧毁敌人的外层空间通信卫星，关闭大部分先进的智能系统。

（5）and 表示对照

例句

Certain materials, such as silver and copper, have many free electrons. <u>And</u> some materials have practically no free electrons.

某些材料，如银和铜，有许多自由电子。<u>而</u>有些材料实际上没有自由电子。

Motion is absolute, <u>and</u> stagnation is relative.

运动是绝对的，<u>而</u>静止是相对的。

（6）and 表示条件

例句

Give me the money <u>and</u> I would buy a new car.

如果给我那笔钱，我会买一辆新车。

Keep your face to the sunshine, <u>and</u> you cannot see your shadow.

如果面对阳光，<u>就</u>看不见自己的影子。

（7）and 表示递进

✔️ 例句

All bodies consist of molecules <u>and</u> these (molecules consist) of atoms.

所有的物体都是由分子组成的，<u>而</u>这些分子是由原子组成的。

In the range of 70~90 dB, speech communication becomes increasingly difficult <u>and</u> eventually impossible.

在 70～90 dB（噪声）范围，对话越来越困难，<u>以至于</u>最后无法进行。

Currently, there exist technologies that hold great promise to expand the capabilities of the health care system, extending its range into the community, improving diagnostics and monitoring, <u>and</u> maximizing the independence and participation of individuals.

目前，存在着一些技术，它们有很大的潜力来提高医疗保健系统的能力，扩大医疗保健系统的范围，改善诊断和监测，最大限度地提高个人的独立性和参与性。

（8）and 表示转折

✔️ 例句

Work sponsored by the British Compressed Air Society showed that in practice the oil density in compressed air is within the range 44 to 72 mg·m^{-3} <u>and</u> in the present work an oil mist/air density of approximately 90 mg·m^{-3} was used as representing a reasonable compromise between typical service conditions and a convenient test duration.

英国压缩空气协会所赞助的研究表明，实际上压缩空气中的油的密度为 44~72 mg·m^{-3}，<u>但是</u>目前实验中采用的浓度约为 90 mg·m^{-3}。这样做是综合考虑了典型的工作环境与适宜的实验时间两个因素。

The parents' attitude and handling of the child is not, of course, the only factor that shape psychological growth. Later in life other people will influence the child's emerging character <u>and</u>, before anyone has a chance to have any effect, inherited traits lay the groundwork for his or her characteristics.

当然，并非只有父母的举止和他们对待孩子的态度是孩子心理发育的影响因素。在以后的生活中，其他人也会影响孩子正在成型的性格。<u>但是</u>在任何人施加任何影响之前，是遗传特性给孩子的性格奠定了基础。

（9）and = with

✔️ 例句

In addition, a plug-in fault diagnostic unit <u>and</u> signal monitoring system is normally supplied with the drive to enable any drive alarm or control signal to be checked and monitored.

此外，一个<u>带有</u>信号监控系统的插入式故障诊断器通常装有传动装置，使任何传动或控制信号得到监控。

（10）and 表示连接对等的人或事物

例句

Biomedical Engineering brings together engineers <u>and</u> clinicians with the aim of improving clinical tools by the application of engineering research, techniques and innovation to the field of clinical medicine.

生物医学工程汇集了工程师<u>和</u>临床医生，目的是通过将工程研究、技术和创新应用到临床医学领域来改进临床工具。

Physiological monitoring could help in both diagnosis <u>and</u> ongoing treatment of a vast number of individuals with neurological, cardiovascular <u>and</u> pulmonary diseases such as seizures, hypertension, dysthymia and asthma.

生理监测可以帮助诊断<u>和</u>治疗大量患有神经、心血管和肺部疾病的人，如癫痫、高血压、心境恶劣症<u>和</u>哮喘。

The biochip contains an integrated biosensor array for detecting multiple parameters <u>and</u> uses a passive microfluidic manipulation system instead of active microfluidic pumps.

该生物芯片包含一个集成的生物传感器阵列，用于检测多个参数，<u>并</u>使用被动微流体操作系统代替有源微流体泵。

2. or

在英语中，or 也是一个极为普遍的连接词，其基本意思是"或，不然，否则，左右"。其实，or 在句中可以有多种特殊用法，表示多种意义。

（1）用以引出另一种可能，表示"或，或者，还是"。

例句

Examples of instrumented environments include sensors and motion detectors on doors that detect opening of, for instance, a medicine cabinet, refrigerator, <u>or</u> the home front door.

仪器化的环境的例子包括位于门上的传感器和运动检测器，它们可以检测到药物柜、冰箱<u>或</u>家门的开启。

This approach has the characteristic of being totally unobtrusive and of avoiding the problem of misplacing <u>or</u> damaging wearable devices.

这种方法具有完全不引人注意的特点且可以避免被放置错误<u>或</u>损坏可穿戴设备等问题。

（2）用于否定，连接提出的两种或多种事物，表示"也不，又不"。

例句

He can't read <u>or</u> write.

他不会读，<u>也不</u>会写。

There are people without homes, jobs <u>or</u> families.

有人既无房屋，又无工作，<u>又无</u>家庭。

（3）用于警告或忠告，表示"否则，不然"。

例句

Turn the heat down <u>or</u> it'll burn.

把炉火开小一些，<u>不然</u>就烧焦了。

（4）用于两个数字之间表示约略数目，译为"大约"。

例句

There were six <u>or</u> seven of us there.
我们<u>约</u>有六七个人在场。

（5）用于引出解释性词语，表示"或者说"。

例句

Geology, <u>or</u> the science of the earth's crust.
地质学，<u>或者说</u>地壳的科学。

It weighs a kilo, <u>or</u> just over two pounds.
这东西重一公斤，<u>或者说</u>两磅多一点儿。

（6）用于说明原因，译为"不然的话"。

例句

He must like her, <u>or</u> he wouldn't keep calling her.
他一定喜欢她，<u>不然的话</u>他不会老给她打电话。

（7）用于引出对比的概念

例句

He was lying—<u>or</u> was he?
他在说谎，<u>还是</u>没有说谎？

10.2   Listening: Bioinstrumentation

Section 1

Bioinstrumentation is a new and upcoming field, concentrating on treating diseases and bridging together the engineering and medical worlds. The majority of innovations within the field have occurred in the past 15~20 years. Bioinstrumentation has revolutionized the medical field, and has made treating patients much easier. The instruments/sensors convert signals found within the body into electrical signals. There are many subfields within bioinstrumentation, which include: biomedical options, creation of sensors, genetic testing, and drug delivery. Other fields of engineering, such as electrical engineering and computer science, are related to bioinstrumentation.

Bioinstrumentation has since been incorporated into the everyday lives of many individuals, with sensor-augmented smart phones capable of measuring heart rate and oxygen saturation, and the widespread availability of fitness apps, with over 40,000 health tracking apps on iTunes alone. Wrist-worn fitness tracking devices have also gained popularity, with a suite of on-board sensors capable of measuring the user's biometrics, and relaying them to an app that logs and tracks information for improvements.

Section 2

Circuits/creation of sensors

Sensors are the most well-known aspect of bioinstrumentation. They include thermometers, brain scans, and electrocardiograms. Sensors take in signals from the body, and amplify them so engineers and doctors can study them. Sensors are amplified using circuits. Circuits take in a voltage source, and modify them using resistors, capacitors, inductors, and other components. They then let out a certain amount of voltage, which is used for analysis. The data collected using sensors is often displayed on computer programs. This field of bioinstrumentation is closely related to electrical engineering.

Biomedical optics

Biomedical optics is the field of performing noninvasive operations and procedures to patients. This has been a growing field, as it is easier and does not require the patient to be opened. Biomedical optics is made possible through imaging such as CAT (computerized axial tomography) scans. One example of biomedical optics is LASIK eye surgery, which is a laser microsurgery done on the eyes. It helps correct multiple eye problems, and is much easier than other surgeries. Other important aspects of biomedical optics include microscopy and spectroscopy.

Section 3

Genetic testing

Bioinstrumentation can be used for genetic testing. This is done with the help of chemistry and medical instruments. Professionals in the field have created tissue analysis instruments, which can compare the DNA of different people. Another example of genetic testing is gel electrophoresis. Gel electrophoresis uses DNA samples, along with biosensors to compare the DNA sequence of individuals. Two other important instruments involved in genomic advances are microarray technology and DNA sequencing. Microarrays reveal the activated and repressed genes of an individual. DNA sequencing uses lasers with different wavelength, to determine the nucleotides present in different DNA strands. Bioinstrumentation has changed the world of genetic testing, and helps scientists understand DNA and the human genome better than ever before.

Drug delivery/aiding machines

Drug delivery and aiding machines have been improved greatly by bioinstrumentation. Pumps have been created to deliver drugs such as anesthesia and insulin. In the past, patients would have to visit doctors more regularly, but with these pumps, they can treat themselves in a faster and cheaper way. Aiding machines include hearing aids and pace makers. Both of these use sensors and circuits, to amplify signals and reveal when there is an issue to the patient.

◆ *Source: https://en.wikipedia.org/wiki/Bioinstrumentation.*

Listening Exercises

Listen to each section twice, and as you are listening, (a) number the words or expressions in the list on the work sheet by order of their first appearance in the passage you are listening to; (b) check if your numbering is correct—if incorrect, listen to the section again; (c) orally answer the questions about the content of each section.

Unit 10, Section 1

biometrics	innovations	treating
creation	saturation	within
everyday	tracks	wrist-worn

1. What are the signals found in the body converted into?

2. Name three of the subfields within the field of bioinstrumentation.

3. How can individuals monitor such things as their heart rate or oxygen saturation as they go about their daily activities?

Unit 10, Section 2

aspect	circuits	noninvasive
axial	closely	spectroscopy
capacitors	electrocardiograms	surgeries

1. What needs to happen to the signals taken from the body so they can be studied by engineers and physicians?

2. What field is closely related to bioinstrumentation?

3. Name one application of bioinstrumentation that is used in a non-invasive type of operation.

Unit 10, Section 3

created	improved	pumps
different	microarray	reveal
genomic	nucleotides	sequencing

1. What kind of instrument can be used for genetic testing?

2. How can activated or repressed genes of a person be revealed?

3. How can drugs such as insulin be administered inexpensively by a patient?

Unit 11　Medical Imaging

11.1　Text: Medical Imaging

Biomedical imaging has revolutionized medicine and biology by allowing us to see inside the body and to visualize biological structure and function at microscopic levels. Images are representations of measurable properties that vary with spatial position (and often time). Images can provide exquisitely detailed information about biological structures; the most powerful imaging modalities provide functional information as well, allowing the recording of molecular or cellular processes, or physical properties (such as elasticity or temperature). Methods to visualize and quantify these properties are now available at the macroscopic (i.e., of a size visible to the human eye) and microscopic level. This information can be used clinically for diagnosis and monitoring of treatment as well as scientifically for understanding normal and abnormal structure and physiology.

Technology has brought about remarkable changes in imaging. Gene expression can now be imaged using positron emission tomography (PET) imaging—an image creation method that depends on injection of special radioisotopes—coupled with methods from genetics.[1] The brain can be imaged at work on cognitive tasks with functional MRI (fMRI)，and that information can be used to guide neurosurgery. The mechanical action of the heart can be mapped using high-frequency sound waves (ultrasound imaging); these maps identify areas of injury after a heart attack. Images are essential tools in medicine because they provide a spatial map, enabling physicians to localize the biological phenomena being examined in space as well as time.

The many different imaging modalities—or types of imaging methods—fill different scientific and/or clinical niches. Every modality has limitations: a particular method may be low in quality, slow to acquire images, expensive, or not suitable for all patients. The set of advantages for a particular technology (e.g., high quality, faster, cheaper, or dynamic) will make it suitable in the right situations. Different modalities operate over different time or length scales and—because of the physics that underlie their operation—can measure different structures or functions.[2] Virtually all imaging modalities are now digital; the images are acquired by a computer and are made up of individual picture elements, or pixels. Digital images can be readily processed to improve their quality, make measurements, and extract features of interest.

Glossary

microscopic [ˌmaɪkrə'skɒpɪk]　　　　*adj.* 微小的，显微镜的
exquisitely [ɪk'skwɪzɪtlɪ]　　　　　*adv.* 剧烈地，异常地

elasticity [ˌiːlæˈstɪsɪti]	n. 弹性，弹力
neurosurgery [ˈnʊrosɜdʒərɪ]	n. 神经外科
macroscopic [ˌmækrəˈskɒpɪk]	adj. 宏观的
radioisotope [ˌɹedioˈaɪsətop]	n. 放射性同位元素
niche [nɪtʃ]	n. 壁龛，合适的位置
pixel [ˈpɪksəl]	n. 像素

Technical Terms

positron emission tomography (PET)	正电子成像术
functional MRI (fMRI)	功能性磁共振成像
imaging modality	显像模式

Notes

1. Gene expression can now be imaged using positron emission tomography (PET) imaging—an image creation method that depends on injection of special radioisotopes—coupled with methods from genetics.

基因表达现在可以用依赖于注入特殊放射性同位素的正电子成像术（PET）结合遗传学方法来成像。

分析：that 引导定语从句，修饰 an image creation method, an image creation method that depends on injection of special radioisotopes 在句中作为 PET imaging 的同位语。

2. Different modalities operate over different time or length scales and—because of the physics that underlie their operation—can measure different structures or functions.

不同的显像模式可以在不同的时间或长度尺度上运作，并且由于操作的物理机制不同，它们可以测量不同的结构和功能。

Translation Skills：否定句的翻译

无论在英语中还是在汉语中，肯定句和否定句都是人们日常交际常用的表达手段和陈述方式。在英语中经常能见到带否定词的短语和习语，有的甚至并不表示否定意愿。下文将列举科技论文中常见的几个带否定词的短语。

at no time	从来没有
by no means (under no circumstances; in no account)	决不
come to nothing	毫无结果
have nothing in common	与……毫无共同之处
make no difference	没有关系，没有影响
more often than not	多半，通常
not a bit	一点也不
not a quarter	远不是，完全不是
not amount too much	没有什么了不起
not to speak of	更不用说，当然

nothing but, nothing else but (than), nothing less than	只不过是，不外是
spare no pains	不遗余力
to say nothing of	更不用说……了
there is no (little) doubt	毫无疑问

由于文化背景、语言习惯和表达方式的不同，英汉两种语言在意义表达上有很大的区别，尤其是在否定句的应用方面。这给学生的理解和翻译造成了很大的障碍。翻译英语否定句，首先要弄清楚其结构及用法上的一些特点，否则就容易出错。

1. 全部否定

全部否定指将句子陈述的对象加以彻底的否定，通常使用一些含"绝无"意义的否定词加上肯定式谓语来表示。这些否定词常以字母"n"开头，如 no、not、none、never、nobody、nothing、nowhere、nor、neither、neither…nor…等。此外，还有一些具有否定含义的短语也常被用来表示全部否定。此类英语否定句一般仍译为汉语否定句。

例句

The value of a computer is <u>not</u> because of it's high price.
计算机<u>不是</u>因为价格贵才有价值。

These problems have <u>no</u> satisfactory explanation.
这些问题<u>尚未</u>有令人满意的解答。

Under <u>no</u> circumstances will human beings abuse biological weapons.
在任何情况下，人类都<u>不应该</u>滥用生化武器。

Methylal does <u>not</u> decomposes into CO and H_2 like formaldehyde.
甲缩醛<u>不像</u>甲醛那样可以分解成 CO 和 H_2。

2. 部分否定

部分否定，是对叙述的内容做部分的而不是全部的否定。部分否定主要是由 all、both、every、many、much、each、often、always 等词与否定词构成，相当于汉语"不全是""不总是""并非都""未必都""不是两个都"之意。这类否定句中的否定词 not 有时和谓语在一起，构成谓语否定。该类否定句在形式上很像全部否定，但实际上是部分否定，在翻译时要特别注意。

例句

<u>Not</u> every automated machine tool can work so productively.
<u>不是</u>每一部自动化机床都能如此高效地运转。

Everybody <u>wouldn't</u> like it.
<u>并不是</u>每个人都会喜欢它。

She <u>does not</u> wholly agree that this skin disease might occur in response to the sunlight.
她<u>并不</u>完全同意这种皮肤病的发病是由太阳照射引起的。

3. 半否定

半否定又称为几乎否定，是指整个句子的意思近于否定。半否定可以由 barely（仅仅，几乎不），hardly（几乎不，简直不），only（只，仅仅），rarely（很少，难得），scarcely（几乎没有，简直不），seldom（不常，很少），little 和 few（少，一点儿）等词构成。这些词在意义上是否定的。

例句

I seldom know how to use this meter.
我几乎不会使用这个仪表。

She scarcely seems to care, does she?
她好像没在意，是吗？

4. 双重否定

双重否定句是指在一个句子中连用两个否定词或连用一个否定词与一个表示否定意义的词或词组的句子，如 but、without、absence、fail、keep…from、fall short of 等词或词组的连用。在翻译时，可以照译为汉语中的双重否定，有时也可译为汉语的肯定句，可根据译文及汉语习惯而定。下面介绍几种常用结构的译法。

（1）全否定词+全否定词
当两个全否定词出现在同一句中时构成双重否定。

例句

Without friction, there could be no brake.
没有摩擦就不会有制动。

There are no sound waves unless there is sound.
没有声音，也就没有声波。

Without financial support, the research and development of manned space flights could not be accomplished successfully.
没有资金的支持，载人航天飞机的研发就不能顺利完成。

（2）全否定词+半否定词
当一个全否定词与一个半否定词（few、little、seldom 等）出现在同一句子中时，构成双重否定。

例句

Few students in our college cannot speak English.
我们这个学校几乎没有学生不会说英语。

（3）全否定词+含有否定意义的词
含有否定意义的词主要包括某些带有否定前缀或后缀的单词，如 impossible、unprepared、displeased、disobey 等，以及一些本身含有否定意义的词，如 deny、fail、refuse、neglect、ignore、without 等。

例句

It is <u>no</u> <u>denying</u> the fact that the invention of computer and internet signals the enormous progress in science and technology in the 20th century.

<u>不可否认</u>的是计算机和互联网的发明标志着 20 世纪科学技术的巨大进步。

We shall <u>not</u> <u>fail</u> to help you when necessary.

必要时我们<u>一定会</u>帮助你。

It is <u>not</u> <u>impossible</u> for scientists to seek ways to overcome cancers in the future.

科学家<u>可能</u>在将来找到攻克癌症的方法。

The research team is <u>not</u> <u>unsatisfactory</u> with experimental findings.

研究团队对实验数据<u>不是</u>特别<u>不满意</u>。

（4）全否定词+but

在"全否定词+but"的结构中，but 被用作关系代词，相当于 which/who/that... not...。在该结构中，but 具有否定含义，句子为双重否定句，在译成汉语时要留意其用法。此外，还要注意 nothing (nobody/nowhere/none)...so...but...的双重否定义，这种句子的翻译通常为：无论……只要……就（便）……，……所有（一切）……（只要）……便（就）……。

例句

There is <u>nothing</u> so difficult <u>but</u> it becomes easy by practice.

<u>无论</u>多么困难的事，<u>只要</u>实践便会变得容易。

也可译为：<u>所有（一切）</u>困难的事，<u>只要</u>实践都会变得容易。

5. 意义上的肯定

有些特殊结构的句子形式上是否定的，但意义上是肯定的，这类句子宜翻译为汉语中的肯定句式。例如，含有 no sooner than、no/not/nothing + more/less + than、no less... than、too... not to do...、no... except/until、no +比较级+ than 等结构的句子表达的就是肯定的意思。常见的结构还有：nothing like（没什么比得上……），no/not/nothing + more + than（不过），no/not/nothing + less + than（多达）等。

例句

<u>No less than</u> fifty tons of waste gas are produced in coal-fired power plant.

燃煤电厂在生产过程中可产生<u>多达</u> 50 吨的废气。

The patient could <u>not</u> feel <u>better</u>.

病人感觉<u>很好</u>。

The surgeon can <u>not</u> agree <u>more</u>.

外科医生<u>完全</u>同意。

6. 含蓄否定

含蓄否定句是寓否定意义于肯定表达形式之中的特殊表达方式。从字面上看，这类否定句在形式上是肯定的，但语义却是否定的，有时还特别强烈。在翻译此类句子时，应根据不同的语境译为相应的汉语否定句。

（1）动词或动词短语引起的否定

常见的有 deny（拒绝，否认），fail（失败），lack（缺乏），refuse（拒绝），stop（停止），protect…from（保护……免受），keep…from（避免），overlook（忽视、忽略），miss（失败、错过），等等。

例句

The experiment underlined{failed of} success.
实验没有成功

The value of loss in this equation is so small that we can overlook it.
在此方程中，损耗值太小，可以忽略不计。

The specification lacks detail.
这份说明书不够详尽。

（2）名词引起的否定

常见的有 neglect（忽视），absence（缺乏），loss（失去），exclusion（排除），ignorance（无知），等等。

例句

A few instruments are in a state of neglect.
一些仪器处于无人管理的状态。

（3）形容词或形容词短语引起的否定

常见的有 free from（不受……影响），ignorant of（不知道），short of（缺乏），ast（最不），little（少），few（少），等等。

例句

The precision instrument must be kept free from dust.
精密仪器必须保持无尘。

This equation is underlined{far from} being complicated.
这个方程式一点也不复杂

（4）介词或介词短语引起的否定

常见的有 beyond（超出），above（超出……外），beneath（不值得），beside（同……无关），instead of（而不是），等等。

例句

The problem is beyond the reach of my understanding.
这个问题我无法理解。

The Theory of Relativity worked out by Einstein is now above many people's comprehension.
爱因斯坦提出的相对论，现在还有不少人理解不了。

（5）连词或连词短语引起的否定

常见的有 before（在……以前，尚未……），but（而不），would rather than（宁可……而

不愿，与其……不如），rather than（而不……），too...to（太……不），等等。

 例句

Never start to do the experiment <u>before</u> you have checked the meter.

<u>没有</u>检查好仪表，切勿开始做实验。

11.2　Listening: Medical Imaging

🎧 Section 1

Medical imaging is the technique and process of creating visual representations of the interior of a body for clinical analysis and medical intervention, as well as visual representation of the function of some organs or tissues (physiology). Medical imaging seeks to reveal internal structures hidden by the skin and bones, as well as to diagnose and treat disease. Medical imaging also establishes a database of normal anatomy and physiology to make it possible to identify abnormalities. Although imaging of removed organs and tissues can be performed for medical reasons, such procedures are usually considered part of pathology instead of medical imaging.

As a discipline and in its widest sense, it is part of biological imaging and incorporates radiology which uses the imaging technologies of X-ray radiography, magnetic resonance imaging, medical ultrasonography or ultrasound, endoscopy, elastography, tactile imaging, thermography, medical photography and nuclear medicine functional imaging techniques as positron emission tomography (PET) and single-photon emission computed tomography (SPECT).

🎧 Section 2

Measurement and recording techniques which are not primarily designed to produce images, such as electroencephalography (EEG), magnetoencephalography (MEG), electrocardiography (ECG), and others represent other technologies which produce data susceptible to representation as a parameter graph vs. time or maps which contain data about the measurement locations. In a limited comparison these technologies can be considered as forms of medical imaging in another discipline.

Up until 2010, 5 billion medical imaging studies had been conducted worldwide. Radiation exposure from medical imaging in 2006 made up about 50% of total ionizing radiation exposure in the United States.

Medical imaging is often perceived to designate the set of techniques that noninvasively produce images of the internal aspect of the body. In this restricted sense, medical imaging can be seen as the solution of mathematical inverse problems. This means that cause (the properties of living tissue) is inferred from effect (the observed signal). In the case of medical ultrasonography, the probe consists of ultrasonic pressure waves and echoes that go inside the tissue to show the internal structure. In the case of projectional radiography, the probe uses X-ray radiation, which is absorbed at different rates by different tissue types such as bone, muscle and fat.

The term noninvasive is used to denote a procedure where no instrument is introduced into a patient's body which is the case for most imaging techniques used.

🎧 Section 3

Imaging modalities

(a) The results of a CT scan of the head are shown as successive transverse sections. (b) An MRI machine generates a magnetic field around a patient. (c) PET scans use radiopharmaceuticals to create images of active blood flow and physiologic activity of the organ or organs being targeted. (d) Ultrasound technology is used to monitor pregnancies because it is the least invasive of imaging techniques and uses no electromagnetic radiation.

In the clinical context, "invisible light" medical imaging is generally equated to radiology or "clinical imaging" and the medical practitioner responsible for interpreting (and sometimes acquiring) the images is a radiologist. "Visible light" medical imaging involves digital video or still pictures that can be seen without special equipment. Dermatology and wound care are two modalities that use visible light imagery. Diagnostic radiography designates the technical aspects of medical imaging and in particular the acquisition of medical images. The radiographer or radiologic technologist is usually responsible for acquiring medical images of diagnostic quality, although some radiological interventions are performed by radiologists.

Listening Exercises

Listen to each section twice, and as you are listening, (a) number the words or expressions in the list on the work sheet by order of their first appearance in the passage you are listening to; (b) check if your numbering is correct—if incorrect, listen to the section again; (c) orally answer the questions about the content of each section.

Unit 11, Section 1

abnormalities	pathology	representations
diagnose	positron	single-photon
function	removed	ultrasonography

1. Name two kinds of purposes for which the visual representation of the interior of a body can be used.

2. How can a database of normal anatomy and physiology be used?

3. Name three technologies that could come under the heading of medical imaging.

Unit 11, Section 2

aspect	inverse	parameter
denote	ionizing	projectional
inferred	magnetoencephalography	worldwide

1. Name three measurement and recording techniques that produce data rather than images.

2. What share in worldwide radiation exposure of humans comes from medical imaging?

3. Explain how medical imaging can be seen as the solution of mathematical inverse problems.

Unit 11, Section 3

acquiring	dermatology	pregnancies
acquisition	generates	radiopharmaceuticals
blood flow	practitioner	successive

1. What is the active principle in an MRI?

2. How does a PET scan work?

3. Where is visible light imaging used?

11.3　Writing: Discussion

讨论（discussion）的重点在于对研究结果的解释和推断，并要说明作者的结果是否支持或反对某种观点、是否提出了新的问题或观点等。因此，在撰写讨论时要避免模糊、含蓄，尽量做到直接、明确，以便审稿人和读者了解论文为什么值得关注。

讨论的内容

1．回顾研究的主要目的或假设，并探讨得到的结果是否符合原来的期望。如果与期望不符，需说明原因。

2．概述最重要的结果，并指出该结果是否能支持先前的假设以及是否与其他学者的结果相一致。如果不是的话，需解释说明。

3．对结果提出说明、解释或假设。论述根据这些结果，能得出哪些结论或推论。

4．指出研究的限制以及这些限制对研究结果的影响，并建议进一步的研究题目或方向。

5．指出结果的理论意义（支持或反驳相关领域中现有的理论、对现有理论的修正）和实际应用价值。

具体的写作要求

1．对结果的解释要重点突出，简洁、清楚。为有效地回答研究问题，可适当简要地回顾研究目的并概括主要结果，但不能简单地罗列结果，因为对结果的概括是为"讨论"服务的。

2．推论要符合逻辑，避免实验数据不足以支持观点和结论。在根据结果进行推论时要遵循适度原则，在论证时一定要注意结论和推论的逻辑性。在探讨实验结果或观察事实的相互关系和科学意义时，无须得出试图去解释一切的不符合实际的结论。如果把数据外推从而得到一个更大的、不恰当的结论，不仅无益于提高作者的科学贡献，甚至会导致现有数据所支持的结论被怀疑。

3．观点或结论的表述要清楚、明确。尽可能清楚地指出作者的观点或结论，并解释该结论是支持还是反对早先的工作。在结束讨论时，避免使用诸如 "Future studies are needed." 之类的苍白无力的句子。

4．对结果的理论意义和实际应用价值的表达要实事求是，并适当留有余地。避免使用 for the first time 等类似的优先权声明。在讨论中应选择适当的词汇来区分推测与事实。例如，可选用 prove、demonstrate 等词语来表示作者坚信观点的真实性；选用 show、indicate、find 等词语来表示作者对问题的答案有某些不确定性；选用 imply、suggest 等词语来表示推测；选用情态动词 can、will、should、may、could 等来表示论点的确定性程度。

5．时态的运用可遵循以下几条规则。

（1）回顾研究目的时，通常使用一般过去时。如 in this study, the effects of two different learning methods were investigated。

（2）如果作者认为所概述结果的有效性只是针对本次研究，需用一般过去时；相反，如果结果具有普遍的意义，则用一般现在时。如 the experimental and theoretical values for the yields agree well。

（3）在阐述由结果得出的推论时，通常使用一般现在时。使用一般现在时的理由是作者得出的是普遍有效的结论或推论（而不只是在讨论自己的研究结果），并且结果与结论或推论之间的逻辑关系为不受时间影响的事实。如 the data reported here suggest (these findings support the hypothesis, our data provide evidence) that the reaction rate may be determined by the amount of oxygen available。

6．多使用副标题。可以把讨论分为多个小节并在每个小节前面加一个副标题。如此一来，既可以增加论文的可读性，又能吸引读者的注意力。副标题可以指引读者更轻易地找到自己想阅读或重读的部分。在写副标题时，应注意下面两点：a）副标题至少包含一个名词，不要把单一的形容词当作副标题；b）副标题应该提供具体的信息。应避免使用如 Part I 这种一般的副标题，而应采用如 Reaction Rate 或 Dependence of Reaction Rate on Temperature 或者 Increase in Reaction Rate with Temperature 这种能提供具体信息的副标题。

典型的讨论章节

典型的讨论章节包括下列 6 个项目。

1．研究目的。作者再次指出自己研究的主要目的或假设。

2．结果概述。作者概述最重要的结果，并指出这些结果是否能支持原来的假设及是否和其他学者的结果相一致。有时候，作者还会再次指出个别重要的结果。

3．对于结果的说明。作者对自己的结果提出说明、解释或假设。

4．推论或结论。作者指出自己的研究结果所能支持的较为广泛的推论或结论。

5．研究方法或结果的限制。作者指出自己研究的局限性以及这些局限性对于研究结果的影响。

6．建议新的研究题目或指出研究结果的实际应用价值。

有不少研究报告的讨论章节以上述六个项目为基本的组织结构。然而，也有不少作者并没有直接按照上面的顺序排列。某一篇特定的研究报告可能会省略其中一两个项目，而且，项目 2、3、4 可能会多次重复或可能会穿插进行。

实例

以下讨论章节反映了上述的组织结构。

An Experimental Study on Integrating Formal and Functional Approaches to Language Teaching

研究目的
研究概述

This experimental study was designed to examine the effectiveness of one approach to integrating grammar into a French immersion curriculum. The findings indicate that classes which experienced an approach that integrated formal analytic and functional, communicative activities in writing had better performance than those classes that did not experience this approach. Statistically significant differences were not revealed in speaking. However, an examination of the individual class data revealed greater and more consistent growth in speaking in the experimental than in the control classes, suggesting that they benefited somewhat from the experimental treatment in this area as well.

研究结果
的说明

The relatively smaller gains made by students in speaking than in writing may be attributed to several factors. Among these are the commonly observed lag between assimilation of a new rule and its automatization in speaking (James, 1980), as well as the competition provided by previously automatized rules in the learner's grammar. Detailed error analyses of the speaking data revealed the presence of interlanguage forms...

结论或
推论

Overall, the findings of this study suggest that improvement of students' oral and written grammatical skills can be achieved through curricular intervention that integrates formal analytic and functional, communicative approaches in language teaching. Because of the consistency of the results for the experimental classes, we think that this integrated approach hold much promise for the improvement of language teaching in immersion programs...The speaking results, however, suggest that more time and effort may be needed to allow students to fully assimilate their new grammatical learning...

建议其他
研究题目

This study cannot help resolve the theoretical debate on the importance of production in second-language learning (see Krashen, 1981 and Swain, 1985). Nor could the study isolate the effects of the various instructional features of the experimental materials. This information is important and would contribute to our understanding of both theoretical and practical issues in second-language learning, but one should not preclude the possibility that the key to improve second-language performance in the classroom may lie in the totality of the individual instruction features rather than in their isolation...

This research makes a step toward developing an effective approach for integrating grammar into French classroom. More research is called for concerning the effectiveness of the techniques used in this approach, if possible in teaching other aspects of grammar. In addition, there is a critical need for observational research in immersion classrooms so that effective strategies currently being used by teachers to promote grammatical proficiency can be identified.

Unit 12 Moral and Ethical Issues

12.1 Text: Moral and Ethical Issues

The tremendous infusion of technology into the practice of medicine has created a new medical era. Advances in material science have led to the production of artificial limbs, heart valves, and blood vessels, thereby permitting "spare-parts" surgery. Numerous patient disorders are now routinely diagnosed using a wide range of highly sophisticated imaging devices, and the lives of many patients are being extended through significant improvements in resuscitative and supportive devices such as respirators, pacemakers, and artificial kidneys.

These technological advances, however, have not been entirely benign. They have had significant moral consequences. Provided with the ability to develop cardiovascular assist devices, perform organ transplants, and maintain the breathing and heartbeat of terminally ill patients, society has been forced to reexamine the meaning of such terms as death, quality of life, heroic efforts, and acts of mercy, and consider such moral issues as the right of patients to refuse treatment (living wills) and to participate in experiments (informed consent).[1] As a result, these technological advances have made the moral dimensions of health care more complex, and have posed new and troubling moral dilemmas for medical professionals, biomedical engineers, and society at large.

Technology and ethics are not foreigners; they are neighbors in the world of human accomplishment. Technology is a human achievement of extraordinary ingenuity and utility and is quite distant from the human accomplishment of ethical values. They face each other, rather than interface. The personal face of ethics looks at the impersonal face of technology to comprehend technology's potential and its limits. The face of technology looks to ethics to be directed to human purposes and benefits.

In the process of making technology and ethics face each other, it is our hope that individuals engaged in the development of new medical devices, as well as those responsible for the care of patients, will be stimulated to examine and evaluate critically "accepted" views and to reach their own conclusions.[2]

For biomedical engineers, an increased awareness of the ethical significance of their professional activities has also resulted in the development of codes of professional ethics. Typically consisting of a short list of general rules, these codes express both the minimal standards to which all members of a profession are expected to conform and the ideals for which all members are expected to strive.[3] Such codes provide a practical guide for the ethical conduct of the profession's practitioners. Two moral norms have remained relatively constant across the various moral codes and oaths that have been formulated for health care providers since the beginnings of Western medicine in classical Greek civilization. They are beneficence, the provision of benefits, and nonmaleficence, the avoidance of doing harm.[4]

◆ *Source: Introduction to biomedical engineering.*

Glossary

ethical [ˈeθɪkəl]	*adj.* 伦理学的
infusion [ɪnˈfjuːʒən]	*n.* 投入
resuscitative [rɪˈsʌsəˌteɪtɪv]	*adj.* 苏醒的
respirator [ˈrespɪreɪtə]	*n.* 呼吸机
pacemaker [ˈpeɪsˌmeɪkə]	*n.* 起搏器
benign [bɪˈnaɪn]	*adj.* 良性的
practitioner [prækˈtɪʃənə]	*n.* 实践者；执业医生
ingenuity [ˌɪndʒəˈnjuːəti]	*n.* 独创性，设计新颖
oath [əʊθ]	*n.* 誓言，誓约
beneficence [bɪˈnefɪsəns]	*n.* 行善，仁慈
nonmaleficence [nɒnməˈlefɪsəns]	*n.* 不伤害

Technical Terms

heart valve	心脏瓣膜
blood vessel	血管
dimensions of health care	医疗服务范畴
moral code	道德准则

Notes

1. Provided with the ability to develop cardiovascular assist devices, perform organ transplants, and maintain the breathing and heartbeat of terminally ill patients, society has been forced to reexamine the meaning of such terms as death, quality of life, heroic efforts, and acts of mercy, and consider such moral issues as the right of patients to refuse treatment (living wills) and to participate in experiments (informed consent).

如今，人类已经能够开发心血管辅助装置，实施器官移植，以及维持晚期病人的呼吸和心跳。这迫使人们不得不重新审视死亡、生存质量、英雄壮举及怜悯之心等概念的含义，并且开始考虑病人拒绝治疗的权利（即预立遗嘱）和参与临床实验的权利（即知情同意）。

2. In the process of making technology and ethics face each other, it is our hope that individuals engaged in the development of new medical devices, as well as those responsible for the care of patients, will be stimulated to examine and evaluate critically "accepted" views and to reach their own conclusions.

在科学技术与伦理学相互对峙的过程中，我们希望从事医疗设备开发和负责病人护理的人员能够批判性地审视所谓的"公认"的观点，并总结出自己的观点。

分析：that 引导宾语从句，as well as 并列连接从句的两个主语。

3. Typically consisting of a short list of general rules, these codes express both the minimal standards to which all members of a profession are expected to conform and the ideals for which all members are expected to strive.

这些准则一般由数条规则组成，它们既表明了所有专业人士都应该遵守的最低标准，也指出了所有专业人士都应该追求的目标。

分析：both…and 并列连接两个宾语。to which 引导定语从句，修饰 the minimal standards。

4. They are beneficence, the provision of benefits, and nonmaleficence, the avoidance of doing harm.

行善就是提供帮助，不伤害就是避免伤害。

Translation Skills：复杂句的翻译

1. 增译法

增译法是为了满足读者需求，补充翻译内容的一种方法。由于英汉两种语言具有不同的文化基础、语言习惯和表达方式，在翻译时，为了使译文更符合目标语的语言习惯，译文需要增添一些词、短语或句子，以便更准确地表达原文的意义。使用增译法，既能够保证译文语法结构完整准确，又能够保证译文意思明确清晰。

例句

There has been a growing interest in the development of self-contained lab-on-a-chip systems.
人们对自包含芯片实验室系统的开发越来越感兴趣。

Such systems can revolutionize point-of-care medical testing and diagnosis by making testing and diagnosis fast, cheap and easily accessible.
这种系统可以通过使测试和诊断更快速、更廉价、更普及，进而颠覆性地改变针对性医疗检测和诊断。

Imaging during a breast cancer lumpectomy, for example, allows surgeons to remove the small "breadcrumbs" of cancer that are often left behind, significantly reducing the risk of recurrence.
例如，乳腺癌根治术中的影像检查可以帮助外科医生移除经常被留下的微小的"面包屑"，从而大大降低复发的风险。

The GPS design originally called for 24 SVs, eight each in three approximately circular orbits, but this was modified to six orbital planes with four satellites each.
全球定位系统需要 24 个航天器，有 3 条近似圆形的轨道，每条轨道上有 8 个航天器。但是这种方法后来被改良为使用 6 条轨道，每条轨道上放置 4 个航天器。

2. 省译法

省译法是指在不改变原文意思的基础上，省略原文中部分语句或文字，使译文更加简洁明了。实际上，省译法是删减一些可有可无的，或者在翻译出来之后会违背目标语表达习惯的一些词或短语。但省译并不能删减原文的重要思想，运用省译法是为了达到化繁为简的目的。

✔️**例句**

The yaw-checking ability <u>of the vessel</u> is a measure of the response to counter-rudder applied in a certain state of turning.

偏转抑制能力表示在一定回旋状态下对反舵的响应。

The weight ton of the cargo is the same as the displacement ton and the deadweight ton in the case of a ship, but the measurement ton of cargo is only 40 cubic feet <u>as compared with</u> 100 in the case of ship.

货物的重量吨与船舶的排水吨、载重吨相同，但其容积吨仅为 40 立方英尺，船舶容积吨为 100 立方英尺。

3. 转换法

转换法是指在翻译过程中，为了使译文符合目标语的表述方式和习惯而对原句中的词类、句型和语态等进行转换的方法。具体来说，就是在词性方面，把名词转换为代词、形容词、动词；把动词转换成名词、形容词、副词、介词；把形容词转换成副词和短语。在句子成分方面，把主语变成状语、定语、宾语、表语；把谓语变成主语、定语、表语；把定语变成状语、主语；把宾语变成主语。在句型方面，把并列句变成复合句，把复合句变成并列句，把状语从句变成定语从句。在语态方面，可以把被动语态变为主动语态。

✔️**例句**

Today, movement sensors are <u>inexpensive</u>, <u>small</u> and require very little power, making them highly attractive for patient monitoring applications.

如今，运动传感器<u>价格低廉</u>、<u>体积小</u>、功率极小，因此非常适合用于监护患者的应用软件中。

Remote <u>monitoring</u> of patient status and self-management of chronic conditions represent the most often pursued applications of AAL technologies.

远程<u>监测</u>患者状况和对慢性病的管理是 AAL 技术最常见的应用。

4. 拆句法

拆句法是把一个长而复杂的句子拆译成若干较短、较简单的句子，通常用于英译汉。在英译汉时常常要在原句的关系代词前、关系副词前、主谓连接处、并列或转折连接处、后续成分与主体的连接处，以及意群结束处将长句切断，译成汉语分句。这样就可以基本保留英语语序，顺译全句，同时顺应现代汉语长短句相替、单复句相间的句法修辞原则。

✔️**例句**

I wish to thank you for the incomparable hospitality <u>for which</u> the Chinese people are justly famous throughout the world.

我要感谢你们无与伦比的盛情款待。中国人民正是以这种热情好客而闻名世界的。

We chose to focus on these technologies <u>because</u> recent developments in wearable sensor systems have led to a number of exciting clinical applications.

我们选择专注于这些技术，是因为可穿戴传感器系统的最新进展已带动了许多振奋人心的临床应用的产生。

5. 正译法和反译法

这两种方法通常用于汉译英，偶尔也用于英译汉。所谓正译，是指把句子按照与汉语相同的语序或表达方式译成英语。所谓反译则是指把句子按照与汉语相反的语序或表达方式译成英语。采用正译法与反译法译出的句子常常具有同义的效果，但是用反译法译出的句子往往更符合英语的表达方式和表达习惯。

汉译英：

例句

在美国，人人都能买到枪。

In the United States, <u>everyone</u> can buy a gun. （正译）

In the United States, <u>guns</u> are available to everyone. （反译）

你可以从互联网上获得这一信息。

<u>You</u> can obtain this information on the Internet. （正译）

<u>This information</u> is accessible/available on the Internet. （反译）

他突然想到了一个新主意。

Suddenly <u>he</u> had a new idea. （正译）

<u>He</u> suddenly thought of a new idea. （正译）

<u>A new idea</u> suddenly occurred to/struck him. （反译）

他仍然没有明白我的意思。

He still <u>could not</u> understand me. （正译）

Still he <u>failed to</u> understand me. （反译）

无论如何，她算不上一位思维敏捷的学生。

She can <u>hardly</u> be rated as a bright student. （正译）

She is <u>anything but</u> a bright student. （反译）

英译汉：

例句

Please <u>withhold</u> the document for the time being.

请暂时扣下这份文件。（正译）

请暂时不要发送这份文件。（反译）

6. 包孕法

这种方法多用于英译汉。所谓包孕是指在把英语长句译成汉语时，把英语后置成分按照汉语的正常语序放在中心词之前，使修饰成分在汉语句中形成前置包孕。但修饰成分不宜过长，否则会造成语言拖沓或引发歧义。

例句

A major challenge in biology is to make sense of the enormous quantities of sequence data and structure data <u>that are generated by</u> genome—sequencing projects, proteomics, and other large-scale molecular biology efforts.

生物学的一个主要挑战在于理解测序工程、蛋白质组学和其他规模分子生物研究<u>产生的</u>海量序列数据和结构数据。

You are the representative of a country and of a continent <u>to which China feels particularly close</u>.

您是一位来自<u>使中国倍感亲切的</u>国家和大洲的代表。

What brings us together is that we have common interests <u>which transcend those differences</u>.

使我们走到一起的，是我们有<u>超越这些分歧的</u>共同利益。

<u>A relevant application in the field of rehabilitation</u> relates to the identification of a patient's patterns of activity and on providing suggestions concerning specific exercises.

<u>康复领域的相关应用软件</u>涉及确定患者的活动模式，并针对锻炼情况提出建议。

Accordingly, <u>an individual undergoing monitoring</u> who suffers from, for instance, chronic obtrusive pulmonary disease could receive feedback about not overexerting himself/herself and the performance of rehabilitation exercises that would be prescribed in order to maintain a satisfactory functional level.

因此，<u>正在接受监测的个体患者</u>，如慢性阻塞性肺病患者，可以接收到关于适度训练的建议和患者在规定的康复训练中表现如何的反馈，从而帮助患者保持良好的健康状态。

A wide variety of such signals are commonly encountered <u>in the clinic, research laboratory, and sometimes even at home</u>.

<u>在诊所、研究实验室，有时甚至在家里</u>，都经常会遇到各种各样的该类信号。

7. 插入法

插入法是指把难以处理的句子成分用破折号、括号或前后逗号插入译句中。这种方法主要用于笔译中，偶尔也用于口译中，即用同位语、插入语或定语从句来处理一些解释性成分。

例句

DNA microarray technology, during the past 20 years, has been developed and consolidated as a routine tool in research laboratories and is now transitioning to the clinic.

在过去的 20 年中，DNA 微阵列技术在研究室中已经被开发并整合为常规工具，现在正过渡到诊所。

8. 重组法

重组法是指在进行英译汉时，为了使译文流畅且更符合汉语叙事的习惯，在理清英语长句的结构、明白英语原义的基础上，彻底摆脱原文语序和句子形式，对句子进行重新组合。

例句

Nothing inspired us more [1] as we watched the breathtaking performance of the gymnasts [2] than the final jump of LI Ning [3] that put the Chinese boys on the champion's stand [4].

当我们观看体操运动员惊心动魄的表演时[2]，最鼓舞我们的莫过于李宁的最后一跳[1]+[3]，因为这一跳使得中国男们登上了冠军的领奖台[4]。

In this beautiful golden fall [1], I am very happy [2] to welcome [5] the distinguished guests [7] to

China West Forum 2001 [6] in the ancient capital Xi'an [4], an age-old and mysterious city full of dynamism of the modern era [3].

在美丽的金秋时节[1]，我很高兴[2]能在古老又充满现代活力的[3]古都西安[4]，迎来[5]参加"2001 中国西部论坛"的[6]各位嘉宾[7]。

Decision must be made very rapidly [1]; physical endurance is tested as much as perception [2], because an enormous amount of time must be spent making certain that the key figures act on the basis of the same information and purpose [3].

必须把大量时间花在确保关键人物均根据同一情报和目的行事[3]，而这一切对身体的耐力和思维能力都是一大考验[2]。因此，一旦考虑成熟，决策者就应迅速做出决策[1]。

9. 综合法

综合法是指在单用某种翻译技巧无法译出译文时，着眼篇章，以逻辑分析为基础，同时使用转换法、倒置法、增译法、省译法、拆句法等多种翻译技巧的方法。

例句

People were afraid to leave their houses, for although the police had been ordered to stand by in case of emergency, they were just as confused and helpless as anybody else.

分析：该句共有三层含义：

A. 人们不敢出门；

B. 尽管警察已接到命令，要做好准备以应付紧急情况；

C. 警察也和其他人一样不知所措和无能为力。

在这三层含义中，B 表示让步，C 表示原因，而 A 表示结果。按照汉语习惯顺序，应翻译如下：

尽管警察已接到命令，要做好准备以应付紧急情况，但人们不敢出门，因为警察也和其他人一样不知所措和无能为力。

The phenomenon describes the way in which light physically scatters when it passes through particles in the earth's atmosphere that are 1/10 in diameter of the color of the light.

分析：该句可以分解为四个部分：The phenomenon describes the way [1] in which light physically scatters[2] when it passes through particles in the earth's atmosphere[3] that are 1/10 in diameter of the color of the light [4]. 其中，[1]、[2]和[3]、[4]之间是修饰与被修饰的关系。总体考虑之后，可以使用综合法来翻译这句话，即合译[1]、[2]和[3]，[4]用分译法，这样翻译出来的句子就更符合汉语的表达习惯。

这种现象说明了光线通过地球大气微粒时的物理散射方式。大气微粒的直径为有色光直径的十分之一。

12.2　Listening: Biomedical Engineering Ethics

🎧 Section 1

Biomedical engineers, like all other professionals, are required to abide by certain ethical standards. They are thus expected, not only to keep all applicable laws and regulations, but also to act in the best interest of their clients and society at large. Since they generally work closely with physicians, who rely on their expertise and good judgment, they must remain conscious at all times of the ways in which their techniques and devices used by physicians may affect the lives of patients.

Biomedical engineers work in a vast array of fields, from molecules and cells to artificial organs and limbs, and whatever their specialization, holds a share in the physicians' responsibility. Research and development conducted by biomedical engineers are generally subject to the ethical guidelines and rules adopted by the professional associations of which they are members: honesty is a must; results have to be reported accurately; plagiarism is severely sanctioned, to name only a few of the basic rules.

🎧 Section 2

When animals or humans become research subjects, the researcher must also respect bioethics and medical ethics. In any case the approval of the relevant ethics committee is required before work can begin. Human test subjects must not be harmed in any way. They must give their informed consent before they are allowed to participate. In the case of terminally ill patients on whom an engineered device or procedure is to be tested as a last resort, they must be given full disclosure as to their chance of recovery and possible detrimental effects.

Since biomedical engineering is a relatively new and rapidly diversifying discipline, the development of an ethical framework as well as legislation are bound to lag somewhat behind scientific and technological innovations. The temptation to forge ahead with biomedical engineering projects can be immense when there is any expectation that they may lead to totally novel types of medical intervention, that they may bring huge financial gain and help win the race to a dominant position in national and world markets.

🎧 Section 3

It may be possible to venture into new biomedical and engineering directions without going against the letter of existing ethical codes or breaking the law when there is nothing in the fine print yet stating that a procedure is unethical of illegal. An example might be the creation of designer babies through genetic modification while it is still unclear what the total effect on the human being so created will be and how the subsequently inherited genes will contribute to the future of the human genome. When there is no rule on the books there can be no infraction; when there is no law there can be no crime even when common sense may make people suspect unspecified risks to human life.

And it cannot be assumed that every individual with a high expertise in biomedical engineering is naturally committed to the highest moral principles. It is now common knowledge that engineered performance enhancements to win athletic competitions have been and are still being used, while the perpetrators feel confident that the world will never find out.

Even when researchers are entirely motivated by the desire to help human beings, they may have little power over the ways in which their product is used, as in the case of a life-saving drug, where a speculator acquires the patent for a pittance and then raises the price by more than a thousand percent without ever having contributed a penny towards the research.

◆ *Source: https://ethicsandtechnology.eu/wp-content/uploads/downloadable-content/Brey_2009_Biomed_Engineering.pdf.*

Listening Exercises

Listen to each section twice, and as you are listening, (a) number the words or expressions in the list on the work sheet by order of their first appearance in the passage you are listening to; (b) check if your numbering is correct—if incorrect, listen to the section again; (c) orally answer the questions about the content of each section.

Unit 12, Section 1

abide by	conscious	limbs
array	devices	plagiarism
associations	expertise	responsibility

1. How are biomedical engineers involved in the treatment of patients?
2. Do the insights and decisions of biomedical engineers affect the lives of patients?
3. Who is in charge of the ethical standards of biomedical engineers?

Unit 12, Section 2

consent	diversifying	novel
detrimental	dominant	temptation
disclosure	lag	terminally ill

1. At what stage is the approval of an ethics committee required?
2. Is it ethical to try out a new and so far untested type of medical intervention on a terminally ill patient?
3. What is always required before a medical trial with human participants?

Unit 12, Section 3

committed to	entirely	life-saving
designer	fine print	subsequently
enhancements	infraction	venture

1. Why is it difficult to tell biomedical engineers in complete detail what they are allowed to do?
2. Why do biomedical engineering projects need specialist oversight?
3. Why could a biomedical engineer be tempted to break the law?

12.3　Writing: Conclusion

　　作者在论文的最后通常单独用一章对全文进行总结,让读者对全文的重点有深刻的印象。有的论文也在这一章中提出当前研究的不足之处,对研究的前景和后续工作进行展望。应注意的是,结论章节的目的在于叙述结论,而不在于概述论文的所有内容。摘要才是概述论文内容的部分。此外,在撰写结论时,不应涉及前文不曾指出的新事实,也不能在结论中重复论文其他章节中的句子,或者叙述其他不重要及与自己研究没有密切联系的内容,以故意把结论拉长。

　　并不是所有科技研究报告都有独立的结论章节,在很多领域中,作者都习惯在讨论(discussion)章节中表达所有重要结论,而省略结论章节。然而,在决定是否应包含独立的"结论"章节之前,作者应先参阅自己打算投稿的期刊中曾刊登的研究论文,以推定在自己专业领域中,一般的研究报告是否包含结论章节。

　　如果论文既包含讨论章节又包含结论章节,则结论章节应该相当简短,而且只要简略、清楚地陈述作者研究的两三个主要结论即可。千万不要让读者重读论文其他章节中已表达清楚的资料。

在结论章节中常出现的主要内容

　　结论章节常包括以下内容。

1. 概述论文主要的研究活动(此项可有可无)。
2. 陈述研究的主要结论。这部分可能会包括:
   - 简略地重复最重要的结果;
   - 指出结果的重要意义;
   - 对结果提出可能的说明。
3. 对研究的前景和后续工作的展望(此项可有可无)。

Acknowledgements（致谢）

　　作者可以在论文末尾对他人给予自己的指导和帮助表示感谢,即致谢。致谢一般置于结论之后、参考文献之前,其基本形式为:致谢者+被致谢者+原因。

　　例如,J. Ma is very grateful to the National Science Foundation of China (NNSFC) for the support。

　　也可以具体指出某人做了什么工作使研究工作得以完成,从而表示谢意。

　　如果作者既要感谢某机构、团体、企业或个人的经济资助,又要感谢他人的技术、设备支持,则应按惯例先对经济资助表示感谢,再对技术、设备支持表示感谢。

　　致谢的文字表达要朴素、简洁,以显示其严肃和诚意。

References（参考文献）

　　关于参考文献的内容和格式,建议作者在把握参考文献注录基本原则的前提下,参阅所投刊物的"投稿须知"中对参考文献的要求,或同一刊物的其他论文参考文献的注录格式,确保自己论文的文献列举和标注方法与所投刊物一致。这里只对基本规则做简单介绍。

ISO 5966-1982 中规定参考文献应包含以下三项内容：作者、题目、有关出版事项。其中，出版事项包括书刊名称、出版地点、出版单位、出版年份，以及卷、期、页等。

参考文献的具体编排顺序有以下两种：

- 按作者姓氏字母顺序排列（alphabetical list of references）；
- 按序号编排（numbered list of references），即对各参考文献按引用的顺序编排序号，正文中引用时只要写明序号即可，无须列出作者姓名和出版年份。

目前常用的正文和参考文献的标注格式有三种。

① MLA 参考文献格式。MLA 参考文献格式由美国现代语言协会（Modern Language Association）制定，适合人文科学类论文，其基本格式是在正文中标注参考文献作者的姓和页码，在文末单列参考文献项，以 Works Cited 为标题。

② APA 参考文献格式。APA 参考文献格式由美国心理学会（American Psychological Association）制定，多适用于社会科学和自然科学类论文，其基本格式为是正文引用部分注明参考文献作者姓氏和出版时间，在文末单列参考文献项，以 References 为标题。

③ Chicago 参考文献格式。该格式由芝加哥大学出版社（University of Chicago Press）制定，可用于人文科学类和自然科学类论文，其基本格式是在正文中按引用先后顺序连续编排序号，在该页底以脚注（footnotes）或在文末以尾注（endnotes）的形式注明出处，或在文末单列参考文献项，以 Bibliography 为标题。

其他

1．Appendix（附录）

附录主要包括冗长定理的证明，以及实验中装置的冗长描述及参数等。

2．Notes（注释）

注释用于补充说明正文中某些需要解释但不适合在正文中叙述的内容。注释可以为脚注或尾注形式，其内容可包括相关背景、人物、专有名称的解释，也可作为参考文献的一种列写形式。当以后者形式出现时，其书写形式遵循参考文献注录的基本格式，只是每一条注释都应有编号。

3．Notation/Nomenclature（符号或术语）

有些刊物要求论文作者将文中出现的各种符号、希腊字母所代表的含义单独列出，并标明为 Notation 或 Nomenclature，以便读者参阅。该部分一般放在正文之后、参考文献之前，也有的放在引言之后，甚至可能不出现 Notation 或 Nomenclature 字样，只用一方框列出具体内容，而通用符号可以不解释。

Appendix: Answers to Listening

Unit 1, Section 1

bioengineering 1	monitoring 3	regenerative 9
decommissioning 5	procurement 4	spanning 7
interdisciplinary 6	prostheses 8	therapeutic 2

Unit 1, Section 2

bioartificial 8	hepatic 9	tracheae 7
bioinformatics 1	organelles 2	transplants 6
construct 3	sensing 4	via 5

Unit 1, Section 3

category 1	dialysis 6	mitigation 4
confronted 9	implementation 8	predominantly 2
diagnosis 3	infusion 5	somato 7

Unit 2, Section 1

interdisciplinary 1	nucleotide 7	queries 4
interpret 2	organizational 8	repeatedly 6
methodology 5	proteomics 9	silico 3

Unit 2, Section 2

analysis 5	catalogue 8	extraction 2
annotating 3	evolutionary 7	ontologies 4
biomolecular 9	expression 6	techniques 1

Unit 2, Section 3

algorithms 8	computationally 7	mitosis 9
cluster 6	implementation 4	pressing 2
computational 3	locate 5	states 1

Unit 3, Section 1

fully-featured 1	keynote speech 7	reporting 9
high resolution 6	peek 5	terminology 4
immersive 2	recommended 8	vessels 3

Unit 3, Section 2

challenging 5	correlations 9	intuitive 8
cognitive 3	distractors 2	range 4
complement 6	gamification 1	textual 7

Unit 3, Section 3

aesthetics 4	grab 2	realistic 1
arterial 6	integumentary 9	skeletal 5
endocrine 8	lymphatic 7	stereoscopic 3

Unit 4, Section 1

biocompatible 9	diagnostic 3	investing 4
biological 7	encompasses 5	suitable 8
chemistry 6	interact 1	therapeutic 2

Unit 4, Section 2

autograft 4	intraocular 5	passive 2
cochlear replacements 7	mesh 9	polymers 1
impregnated 3	nerve conduits 8	prostheses 6

Unit 4, Section 3

ambiguity 7	eventually 9	specific 5
behaviour 4	insights 8	traceability 3
elicit 6	issues 1	undergone by 2

Unit 5, Section 1

applications 9	neuroregeneration 6	plaque 1
capitalize on 7	outfitted 3	somewhat 2
innovation 8	peripheral 5	testament 4

Unit 5, Section 2

analysis 2	established 9	singled out 1
coming into its own 8	quintuple 6	stem cell 4
decades 7	release 5	various 3

Unit 5, Section 3

achievement 6	plastic surgeon 1	steep increase 9
cartilage 3	prominent 5	supported 8
chondrocytes 4	publish 2	targeting 7

Unit 6, Section 1

almost 8	continuum 5	modeling 9
approximations 4	kinematics 6	organelles 2
aspects 1	man-built 7	related to 3

Unit 6, Section 2

array 4	implants 8	perturbations 6
cartilage 9	organisms 3	ranges 1
electromyography 5	orthopaedic 7	soft tissue 2

Unit 6, Section 3

athlete 8	implications 7	reduce 2
executes 9	mechanics 1	stated 6
gauges 4	neurophysiology 5	understand 3

Unit 7, Section 1

adapt 2	design 1	physiatrist 5
amputation 6	interarticular 9	recreational 7
cognition 4	joint 8	trauma 3

Unit 7, Section 2

ability 1	impairment 2	quality of life 8
facilitators 5	optimization 4	re-hospitalization 9
goal setting 6	premorbid 3	towards 7

Unit 7, Section 3

acquired 1	instructed 8	pediatric 5
chronic condition 7	outpatient 6	spinal cord injury 3
inpatient 2	palsy 4	trigger point 9

Unit 8, Section 1

analyte 1	biomimetic 3	principles 9
antibodies 2	electrochemiluminescence 5	results 7
associated 6	physiochemical 4	transducer 8

Unit 8, Section 2

contaminants 4	mycotoxins 9	requirements 1
discovery 8	pathogens 7	spawning 6
disposable 2	remote sensing 5	targets 3

Unit 8, Section 3

blood glucose 1	environmental 9	oxidizes 2
canary 6	enzyme 3	transducer 5
current 4	organisms 7	warn 8

Unit 9, Section 1

beings 1	galvanic 9	subsumed 3
bioelectrical 5	magnetoencephalogram 8	time signals 4
electroencephalogram 6	mechanomyogram 7	time-varying 2

Unit 9, Section 2

acoustic 7	in particular 4	oxygenation 9
breathing 8	measurement 1	remote 3
electric 2	non-electrical 6	resistances 5

Unit 9, Section 3

alignment 7	correspond 5	pertaining 2
ambiguities 6	grouped 4	relevant 3
computational 1	optimum 9	target 8

Unit 10, Section 1

biometrics 8	innovations 2	treating 1
creation 4	saturation 6	within 3
everyday 5	tracks 9	wrist-worn 7

Unit 10, Section 2

aspect 1	circuits 3	noninvasive 6
axial 7	closely 5	spectroscopy 9
capacitors 4	electrocardiograms 2	surgeries 8

Unit 10, Section 3

created 1	improved 7	pumps 8
different 2	micro-array 4	reveal 9
genomic 3	nucleotides 6	sequencing 5

Unit 11, Section 1

abnormalities 4	pathology 6	representations 1
diagnose 3	positron 8	single-photon 9
function 2	removed 5	ultrasonography 7

Unit 11, Section 2

aspect 5	inverse 6	parameter 2
denote 9	ionizing 4	projectional 8
inferred 7	magnetoencephalography 1	worldwide 3

Unit 11, Section 3

acquiring 7	dermatology 8	pregnancies 5
acquisition 9	generates 2	radiopharmaceuticals 3
blood flow 4	practitioner 6	successive 1

Unit 12, Section 1

abide by 1	conscious 3	limbs 6
array 5	devices 4	plagiarism 9
associations 8	expertise 2	responsibility 7

Unit 12, Section 2

consent 1	diversifying 5	novel 8
detrimental 4	dominant 9	temptation 7
disclosure 3	lag 6	terminally ill 2

Unit 12, Section 3

committed to 6	entirely 8	life-saving 9
designer 3	fine print 2	subsequently 4
enhancements 7	infraction 5	venture 1

References

[1] 任胜利. 英文科技论文的写作要点. http://lm2000i.bokee.com/viewdiary.13783737.html.

[2] 万灵. 用英文写作科技论文的一般格式[J]. 黄石高等专科学校学报，2004，20(1)：30-33.

[3] 孙富春. 英文科技论文写作体会. http://jcst.ict.ac.cn/attached/file/20180905/20180905093637-954.pdf.